GERIATRICS, GERONTOLOGY AND ELDERLY ISSUES

THE FUTURE OF LONG-TERM CARE

GERIATRICS, GERONTOLOGY AND ELDERLY ISSUES

Additional books and e-books in this series can be found on Nova's website under the Series tab.

GERIATRICS, GERONTOLOGY AND ELDERLY ISSUES

THE FUTURE OF LONG-TERM CARE

PABLO VILLALOBOS DINTRANS
EDITOR

nova
Medicine & Health
New York

Library of Congress Cataloging-in-Publication Data

ISBN: 978-1-53619-263-6

Published by Nova Science Publishers, Inc. † New York

At a time of COVID-19 when many countries are realizing the particular vulnerability of the older people, this book puts the problem of caring for this group in a broad context across a spectrum of low-, middle- and high-income countries. It presents a variety of approaches to long-term care and shows the need for more information on its actual practice, in order to find appropriate ways to address the health and economic needs of both the people with needs and those who care for them. This book is a must-read for policymakers and academics interested in how to approach long-term care policy but it is also useful for those who will benefit from better ways to provide care.

Thomas J. Bossert
Harvard T.H. Chan School of Public Health

This book is an important step in understanding and demystifying one of the most pressing issues in contemporary society: the provision of long-term care in societies facing demographic changes. The evidence and experiences in countries with a varied socioeconomic and cultural context not commonly published show innovative ways to present their needs and approaches. The book presents challenges, good practices, and solutions in diverse settings, providing important lessons for not just countries with similar conditions, but also so low and middle-income countries can find their own way in dealing with the future increase in long-term care needs.

Enrique Vega
Pan American Health Organization

CONTENTS

Preface		**ix**
Acknowledgments		**xv**
Chapter 1	Long-Term Care: Challenges for a Changing World *Pablo Villalobos Dintrans*	**1**
Chapter 2	The Future of Long-Term Care in Developing Countries: Insights from Turkey *Fatih Cemil Ozbugday and Abdullah Tirgil*	**25**
Chapter 3	The Future of Long-Term Care in the United States *Katherine Swartz and Judy Feder*	**73**
Chapter 4	Towards a Better Understanding of the Long-Term Care Needs of Older People in Ghana *Kofi Awuviry-Newton, Meredith Tavener, Kylie Wales and Julie Byles*	**117**
Chapter 5	Addressing Long-Term Care Financing Challenges in the United Arab Emirates *Ahmed Saleh Al Awlaqi*	**143**

Chapter 6 Towards a Long-Term Care System in Mexico **173**
Emmanuel González-Bautista,
Luis Miguel F. Gutiérrez-Robledo,
Mariana López-Ortega and Eduardo Sosa-Tinoco

Chapter 7 The Long-Term Care Insurance System in South Korea: Overview and Future Challenges **217**
Misook Song and Hyunjong Song

About the Editor **245**

About the Contributors **247**

Index **255**

PREFACE

The demographic change has been shaping the countries around the world for years. One stylized fact today is that population aging will become a major issue in many countries, a process that will continue at an accelerated path particularly in developing nations.

One of the main changes coming with the process of population aging is a global expected increase in long-term care (LTC) needs. This rise in the demand for LTC around the world has no precedent both in terms of speed and scale. The gaps in LTC services existing today in many countries calls for comprehensive and urgent measures: implementing LTC solutions will be one of the main challenges in the coming years.

In this context, this book hopes to contribute to the existing literature on LTC and public policy, providing new insights for a must-needed global debate.

WHY THIS BOOK?

Despite being a research and policy subject for many years now, long-term care research still has a long way to go. There is still a lack of consensus in fundamental issues, from theoretical developments to practical solutions. So far, countries with the most pressing needs—notably those with larger proportion of LTC needs in the population—have been the first ones acting into implementing solutions. They have traveled a road full of self-discoveries and using trial and error approaches. The lack of basic definitions and strategies to deal with LTC needs push them into the seek for idiosyncratic solutions; many of them have solved issues regarding the design and implementation of LTC systems establishing ad hoc solutions.

However, we know that many countries will be looking for strategies to cope with this challenge in the coming years. Learning lessons from other countries is an important step but these countries will need to build their own systems, based not just on their needs, but also their context, values, and lessons from other settings.

Why is this book so necessary today? The literature on LTC is still scarce and—although there are notable exceptions, particularly in most recent years—mostly constrained to OECD/developed countries. Since this is an expected outcome of the previously described process—countries that faced the more pressing need responded first—there are at least two problems with promoting and using this evidence exclusively:

- It contributes to the idea that LTC is a "rich countries' problem". This, in turn, generates a dangerous inertia for the majority of the countries in the world that will have to face this problem in the coming years, without being prepared for it.
- It hinders space for other countries to express their problems and contribute with their own solutions.

Making LTC a global issue and providing space for countries to have their own reflection processes on how to handle the many challenges coming from the increase in LTC needs is not just out of respect but should also be seen as an effective way to pool more lessons and experiences for building a broader knowledge in the field.

Besides the geographically constrained debate, the discussion on LTC and LTC systems has also revolved mainly about LTC financing. This emphasis tends to create a barrier for the debate on other topics that could be more needed for countries in the search of their own LTC solutions, and ignore important topics that will be relevant for every country. The book also aims to highlight the need to adopt a broader perspective when debating about the implementation of LTC systems, particularly if we hope this process should be extended to each country in the world. Using examples from countries with LTC initiatives already in place, the book presents the ongoing challenges and changes in paradigms for LTC services around the world, particularly in terms of providing quality services, ensuring sustainability, and empowering users.

The book draws experiences from seven different countries, with different demographic, economic, and cultural profiles. The examples include efforts to respond to LTC needs in different regions of the world: Mexico and the United States in the Americas, Ghana in Africa, Thailand and the Republic of Korea in Asia, the United Arab Emirates in the Eastern Mediterranean region, and Turkey in Europe.

Structure of the Book

Chapter 1 is written as an introduction and serves as motivation for the rest of the book. It presents the huge demographic and epidemiological changes experienced in the past decades and the enormous changes that will occur particularly in developing countries in the future. The chapter adopts a social security perspective to discuss long-term care, understood as a commonly ignored issue in the public agenda when debating on population aging. In this approach it presents several arguments to support the implementation of national LTC systems, pointing at the need for urgent action in every country. Finally, it identify challenges for countries that currently lack of a LTC system (strategies to promote action toward the implementation of a system), countries that already have a system in place (thinking about new topics and better solution), as well as widespread challenges to be faced by every country, regarding LTC (particularly considering the scenario post COVID-19 pandemic).

In Chapter 2, Fatih Cemil Ozbugday and Abdullah Tirgil explain the current situation of LTC in Turkey, looking at the necessary responses the country should adopt in the coming years. The chapter proposes an economic approach based on demand and supply for LTC services, looking at the expected changes of the factors behind these two forces. The authors present the institutional arrangement currently in place in the country, including the most recent regulations, institutions involved in the LTC system. They also exhibit several LTC statistics, regarding beneficiaries, benefits, providers, and financing of LTC in Turkey. Finally, projection of changes in the demand and supply for LTC services are calculated, as a necessary piece of information for the debate of the future of LTC in the country.

Katherine Swartz and Judy Feder explore some of the current and future issues in the US long-term care “system”. Chapter 3 shows that the current provision of LTC in the country is primarily financed through the health system—mostly via Medicaid—faces several problems, particularly in terms of quality of services and financial incentives to providers, many of which are becoming more relevant after the COVID-19 pandemic. The authors propose several paths in which the system can be reformed in the short run (increasing resources to the system, increasing caregivers´ earnings, enforcing quality standards, and reducing financial incentives between different sources of financing) as a way to build a LTC social health insurance in the long run.

Chapter 4 is devoted to analyzing the situation of LTC in Ghana. Kofi Awuviry-Newton, Meredith Tavener, Kylie Wales and Julie Byles present the situation of an Africa country experiencing a process of rapid aging, highlighting the need to understand the concept of long-term care needs from a multidimensional approach. The chapter shows how care schemes and policies have evolved in the country, from traditional care during the era of colonization to the panorama faced by families in modern Ghana. Today, the country is at a crossroad that requires mancomunated efforts from different actors of the society.

Ahmed Saleh Al Awlaqi reports on the situation of LTC in the Middle East in Chapter 5, particularly the challenges of financing LTC in the United Arab Emirates (UAE). The chapter presents different financing schemes adopted around the world, as well as the current situation of LTC services in the country. Looking at expenditures in healthcare by different functions, it also discusses the current expenditures in LTC in the UAE, and the alternatives to establish a sustainable way to meet the future population's demands.

In Chapter 6, Emmanuel González-Bautista, Luis Miguel F. Gutiérrez-Robledo, Mariana López-Ortega, and Eduardo Sosa-Tinoco discuss the context of LTC in Mexico. The authors present the current situation of LTC in the country, including services and regulation. Using a framework based on "connecting nodes" they propose the design of a future LTC system in Mexico by looking at human (people and competencies), material (financing and infrastructure) and meta (data and information) capital. Finally, they assess the country´s preparedness to implement this system, as well as the next steps needed to move forward the establishment of a LTC system in Mexico.

Chapter 7 presents the current situation regarding long-term care in the Republic of Korea. Mi Sook Song and Hyunjong Song discuss the recent demographic trends in the country that led to the implementation of the national long-term care insurance in 2008. The piece describes the current system in terms of its beneficiaries, benefits, providers, and financing, and identifies future challenges related to the system's coverage and financial sustainability, and quality of services. It also highlights an important issue—users' preferences for LTC schemes and services—and the increasing need to consider people's decision of "aging in place".

ACKNOWLEDGMENTS

First, this book could have not been possible without the generous contribution of each one of the authors. They provide the necessary inputs to make this possible. Authors put their knowledge and experience in describing the situation of long-term care in their countries, as well as identifying the main challenges for the coming years. Hopefully their effort will contribute to fostering a global debate around long-term care and serve as a contribution to strengthen the network of researchers and policymakers working in the field.

Second, the team from Nova Publishers, that provided the means to change ideas into a concrete book.

Finally, my great appreciation for the work of Rachel Klabunde, who read every chapter of the book, and made corrections and comments. The final version is more interesting, readable and enjoyable than would it be without her help.

In: The Future of Long-Term Care
Editor: Pablo Villalobos Dintrans
ISBN: 978-1-53619-263-6

Chapter 1

LONG-TERM CARE: CHALLENGES FOR A CHANGING WORLD

Pablo Villalobos Dintrans*
Programa Centro Salud Pública, Facultad de Ciencias Médicas,
Universidad de Santiago, Santiago, Chile

ABSTRACT

The world is quickly changing. The demographic and epidemiological transitions are posing important challenges to social security in every country. One of the most salient features of this process is the expected increase in long-term care (LTC) needs, i.e., the share of population that will require help from others to perform activities of daily living.

The implementation of LTC systems arises as one alternative to deal with this challenge. Despite the difficulties in designing and implementing LTC, there are many reasons—economic, ethical, political, and legal—for countries to undertake this effort.

Today, many challenges regarding LTC have been identified. First, a large set of countries should begin debating and taking action towards the implementation of LTC systems. On the other hand, countries with systems already in place face issues related to the sustainability and

* Corresponding Author's E-mail: pvillalobos.d@gmail.com.

quality of LTC services. Finally, the COVID-19 pandemic will generate new challenges for LTC around the world.

Countries need to ensure the availability of resources and emphasize the relevance of moving forward in the implementation of policies to respond to the increasing LTC needs in their population.

1. Demographic Change and Population Aging: A Starting Point

The world is changing. We hear this sentence over and over again, in different contexts. While true, the sentence does not catch people's attention, either because it is too vague or because it is too obvious. However, the world *is* constantly changing, and will continue to do so. We can help our audience by better defining what we mean by "change" and why this is relevant. One of the most spectacular changes we have observed over the past century is the demographic change.

Our world, and many countries in it, has been experiencing dramatic changes in relation to population size and structure. In the words of Ronald Lee: "Before the start of the demographic transition, life was short, births were many, growth was slow and the population was young." (Lee, 2003, p. 167).

During the demographic transition, the population moves from a state of high mortality and high fertility to one of low mortality and fertility. These changes produce significant changes in population growth—typically an initial increase, followed by a subsequent decrease—changing both the size of the population and the distribution of ages (Lee, 2011; Bongaarts, 2009). Starting with the Industrial Revolution, the population grew *pari-passu* with income, following Malthus' thesis "That population does invariably increase when the means of subsistence increase" (Malthus, 1798, p. 61). Today, we have seen many countries follow a process that starts with a decline in mortality rates, followed by a decrease in fertility rates. These changes result in an initial increase in population, which then begins to decline, finally generating the stage of so-called "population aging".

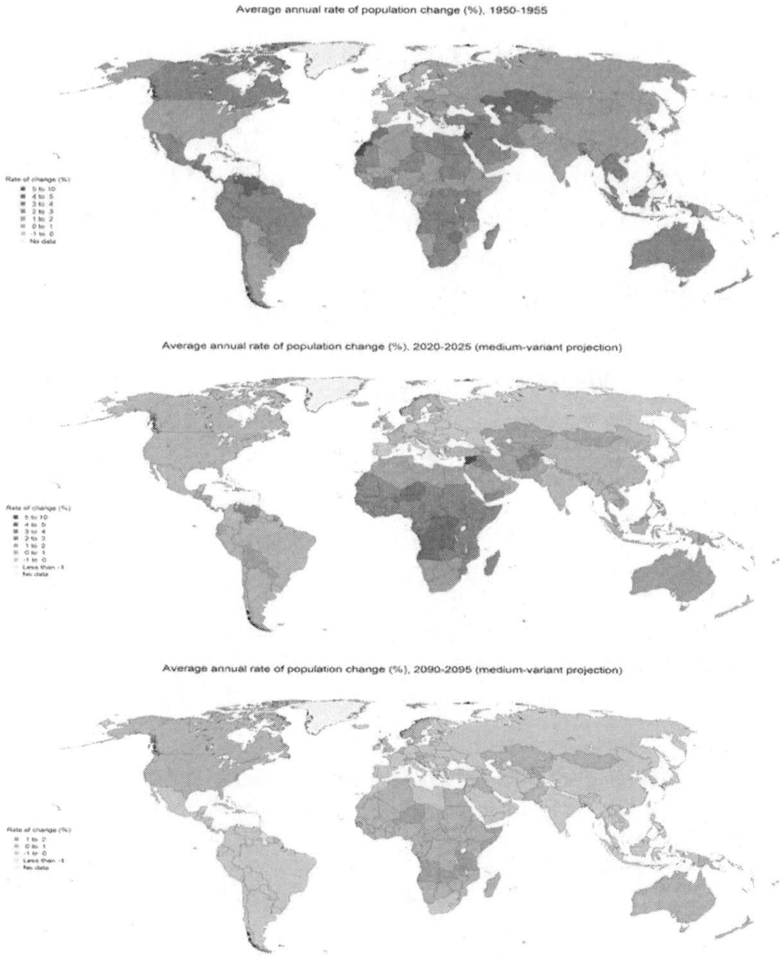

Source: United Nations (2019)

Figure 1. Average annual rate of population change (%) for different periods.

Although countries have experienced similar processes around the world, different places vary with regards to the timing and features of their demographic transition. Broadly speaking, the demographic transition started much earlier and evolved slowly in developed countries, while the process in developing countries is more recent and occurring at an increased pace. For example, data from the United Nations Population Division shows that population growth is slowing at a global level, but this change will continue over decades and differ greatly between countries. Figure 1 shows that 70 years ago (1950), the global population was growing rapidly, with Europe experiencing a more advanced stage in the demographic transition (slow population growth); today, many countries are exhibiting very low growth rates (close to zero), with several countries already experiencing negative growth (population decrease). This trend will continue through the end of the century, although we still observe countries (mostly in Africa) with continuous population growth for the next 70 years.

Similarly, as this occurs, the share of the older population (65+) will increase around the globe. All countries are showing a projected increase in this indicator between 2019 and 2050 (United Nations, 2019); the global share of people aged 65+ will increase from 9% to 23% in 2100. This change will be particularly dramatic in regions like Eastern and South-Eastern Asia and Latin America and the Caribbean. This region, relatively young today, will become the oldest in the world by 2100, with more than 30% of their population in this age group (Table 1).

Table 1. Percentage of population aged 65+ for the world, and SDG regions 2019, 2030, 2050 and 2100, according to the medium-variant projection

Region	**2019**	**2030**	**2050**	**2100**
World	9.1	11.7	15.9	22.6
Sub-Saharan Africa	3.0	3.3	4.8	13.0
Northern Africa and Western Asia	5.7	7.6	12.7	22.4
Central and Southern Asia	6.0	8.0	13.1	25.7
Eastern and South-Eastern Asia	11.2	15.8	23.7	30.4
Latin America and the Caribbean	8.7	12.0	19.0	31.3
Australia/New Zealand	15.9	19.5	22.9	28.6
Oceania*	4.2	5.3	7.7	15.4
Europe and Northern America	18.0	22.1	26.1	29.3

* Excluding Australia and New Zealand.

Source: United Nations (2019).

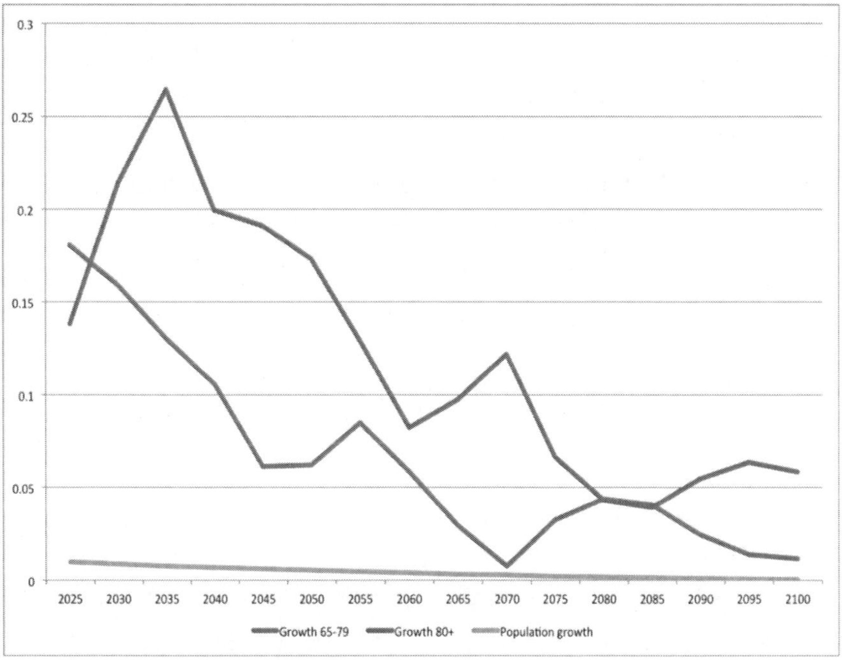

Source: Author elaboration based on United Nations (2019).

Figure 2. Growth rates: total population, population 65-79 and population 80+ in the world.

One of the main differences in this process of population aging for developing regions, compared to the one experienced by regions like Europe and Northern America and Australia/New Zealand, is the short period of time over which significant changes will be produced. As seen in Table 1, countries that today are relatively young will quickly reach the proportion of older population exhibited by developed nations. The speed of aging in these countries has no precedent: while doubling the share of population 65+ (from 10% to 20%) took nearly 70 years in countries like France or Denmark, the same change will occur in less half of the time in countries like Chile, Thailand, or Brazil (United Nations, 2019). This feature represents an important challenge for the majority of countries that will be going through this process of accelerated aging.

Additionally, we observe that not only will the share of older people increase around the world, but the proportion of people 80 years and older will grow particularly quickly. As shown in Figure 2, while population growth will become close to zero, the population between 65 and 70 years will continue increasing at decreasing rates. On the other hand, the people in the age range 80+ will grow at increasing rates for the next 15 years, followed by a decrease in its rate of growth. Nevertheless, the number of people 80+ will continue growing at a higher rate than the group between 65-79 and the rest of the population.

2. Three Challenges for Social Security: Pensions, Health, and Long-Term Care

The increase in the share of population 65+ means a significant change in the way countries will have to approach public policies to meet their citizens' demands. This process will particularly affect social security systems.

Traditionally, this issue has been analyzed from an economic perspective: the increase in the percentage of older people in these countries will change the ratio of productive vs. unproductive members of the society (Villalobos Dintrans, 2019a). This is what most people understand when the discussion on population aging and dependency is proposed. Under this view, dependency is defined as the ratio between the inactive population (over 65 years and under 15 years) and the working population (between 15 and 64), the age-dependency ratio (Bongaarts, 2009). The problem of population aging here is one of the classic problems of economics: limited resources to meet increasing demands. From a social security perspective, this problem is linked *vis-a-vis* the pension system: how to provide income to the increasing number of people retiring with a decreasing number of people working (United Nations, n.d.).

Second, another branch of social security, the health system, is also impacted by these demographic changes. Together with the process of demographic transition, a process of epidemiologic transition has also been occurring. This process, closely related to demographic and socioeconomic changes, is understood as the changing patterns of mortality, fertility, life expectancy, and leading causes of death, modifying the way we live, get sick, and die (Omran, 1971; McKeown, 2009). One of the most salient features of this process is the shift from infectious to non-communicable diseases (NCDs) as the main cause of the burden of disease in the world.

This pattern is observed, for example, looking at the data from the Global Burden of Disease (GBD) project, collected by the Institute for Health Metrics and Evaluation (IHME). Figure 3 shows the distribution of the global burden of disease—measured by disability-adjusted life years (DALYs)[1]—in 1990 and 2017. As observed, the most evident change between the two periods is the increase in the relevance of NCDs as the main source of DALYs in the world.

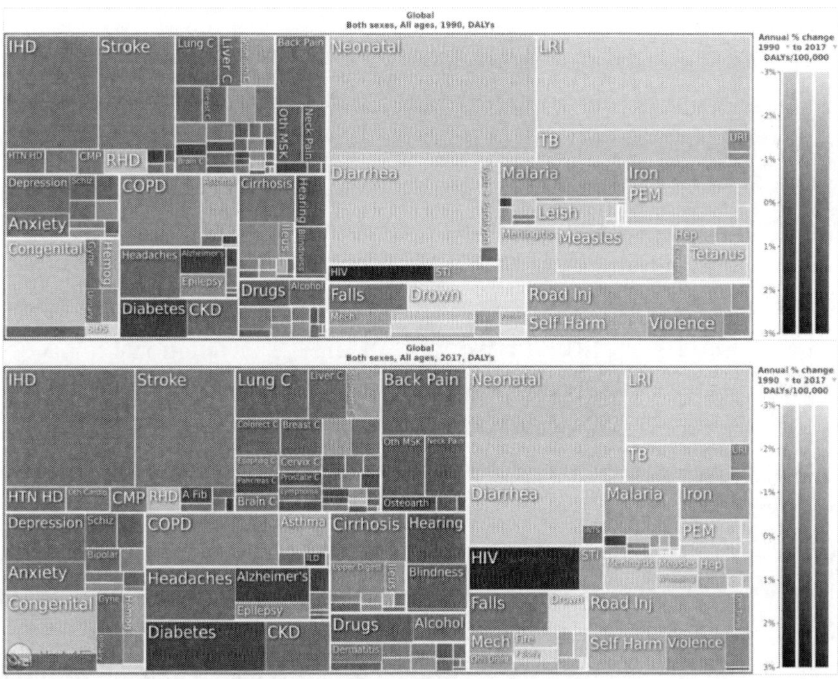

Source: Institute for Health Metrics and Evaluation (2017).

Figure 3. Distribution of global disability-adjusted life years (DALYs), 1990 and 2017.

[1] Disability-adjusted life years (DALYs) is a metric used to compare very different populations and health conditions across time. DALYs equal the sum of years of life lost (YLLs) and years lived with disability (YLDs). One DALY equals one lost year of healthy life (Institute for Health Metrics and Evaluation, 2020).

As in the case of the demographic transition, these changes are not the same for every country. While developed countries have been moving more slowly into this new stage, the changes have been more pronounced in developing countries. Changes in these countries explain the patterns observed in Figure 3. Many of these countries will also experience a double burden of disease, i.e., an increase in the prevalence of NCDs while still dealing with infectious diseases as part of the unfinished agenda in health (World Health Organization, 1999). Changing lifestyles and early life conditions are responsible for this problem, with infectious diseases and NCDs interacting adversely (Bygbjerg, 2012). The demographic and epidemiological transitions introduce an extra challenge to these countries, not just because of the higher burden they face but also because they need stronger health systems to confront these issues (Boutayeb, 2006).

Changes like the new epidemiological profile of the populations and new developments in medicine and public health, together with variations in people's empowerment and their role in their own health, mean that news gaps are created in the supply and demand of healthcare. This could be particularly important for the increasingly larger group of older people. Consequently, several calls have been made recently to adapt the health system to better satisfy the needs of this population (World Health Organization, 2015; 2016). Furthermore, aging has an additional impact on people's finances that should be considered.

So far, we have examined the "traditional issues" arising from population aging. Quoting Victor Fuchs: "In addition to the loss of family and friends and a diminution of status, nearly all older persons face two potentially serious economic problems: declining earning power and increased utilization of health care" (Fuchs, 1999). However, within this debate around population and social security, a new element arises as a required complement to design and implement responses to the previously described challenges: long-term care. Long-term care (LTC) is defined as "activities undertaken by others to ensure that people with a significant ongoing loss of intrinsic capacity can maintain a level of functional ability consistent with their basic rights, fundamental freedoms and human dignity" (World Health Organization, 2015). This concept gives a new meaning to the relationship between population aging and dependency. This "other dependency"—also called care dependency, functional dependency or LTC needs—can be viewed as part of the same discussion (Villalobos Dintrans, 2019a). In this case, however, dependency refers to the need for help in performing everyday activities. Thus, LTC should also be considered as part of a broader debate about social security, in which LTC is usually a missing piece in the system (Villalobos Dintrans, 2018). While pensions are designed to ensure a flow of resources after retiring from the labor force (the income side), health and LTC provide services to maintain and improve living conditions, avoiding an additional financial burden on the people (the expenditure side). As part of the social security system, all these elements should be considered together, since they share important goals and can be used as substitutes (Fuchs, 1999; Villalobos Dintrans, 2018). In the end, money is fungible.

Although demographics is a good starting point for the discussion of LTC, population aging and the increase in LTC needs are not synonyms, although it is true that the increase in LTC needs relates to both the demographic and epidemiologic transitions. It is important to understand these phenomena today, as they allow us to project the likely LTC scenario in the coming years. As noted by Victor Fuchs, "demography is destiny", since the mortality, fertility, size, and age distribution of a population set rigid boundaries for policy makers (2011, p. xii-xiv). This is why demographics are so useful as an umbrella for the discussion on LTC. However, it is important to note that, although age and LTC needs are related (for example, prevalence and severity of LTC needs increase with age (Manton and Stallard, 1994; Freedman et al., 2008; Colombo et al., 2011; Carrera et al., 2013)), LTC is not exclusive to older people (World Health Organization, 2015; Villalobos Dintrans, 2018; 2020).

3. Why Long-Term Care is Important: Different Perspectives

Acknowledging these trends, the World Health Organization (WHO) and other international institutions have made a call to countries around the world to be prepared to face the many challenges of the demographic and epidemiological transitions. In its Global Strategy and Action Plan on Ageing and Health (World Health Organization, 2016), the WHO defined five strategic objectives for dealing with this new reality and promote healthy aging, pointing to "A world in which everyone can live a long and healthy life":

(i) Commitment to action on Healthy Ageing in every country.
(ii) Developing age-friendly environments.
(iii) Aligning health systems to the needs of older populations.
(iv) Developing sustainable and equitable systems for providing long-term care (home, communities and institutions).
(v) Improving measurement, monitoring and research on Healthy Ageing.

Although all objectives are important to fulfill the proposed vision, objective (iv) is directly linked to LTC. The organization, recognizing the future increase in the demand for LTC services worldwide, makes a call for the establishment of LTC systems in every country. Systems of LTC are defined as national systems that ensure integrated LTC is appropriate, affordable, accessible, and upholds the rights of people and caregivers alike (World Health Organization, 2015).

However, the task of designing and implementing national LTC systems is not easy. The LTC system requires making several decisions in terms of financing, coverage, benefits, and needs to complement the other branches of the social security system (Ikegami and Campbell, 2002; Villalobos Dintrans, 2018; 2020). In addition to the technical complexities, the process also needs to sort out political issues. Under this scenario, the call for implementing LTC systems seems like a difficult task. Why should countries embark in this endeavor?

There are several dimensions that justify the need for implementing an LTC system in any country. First, the need to provide solutions for people that currently face the burden of LTC by themselves. The core of the definition of LTC is exactly that: helping people live their lives with dignity. LTC systems have been introduced around the world with this idea in mind. They should be considered a necessary component of social security, since they help protect citizens from a burden that cannot be borne by families or solved by the private sector (Geraedts et al., 2000; Mot, 2010).

From an economic point of view, the implementation of an LTC system can be justified as a strategy for cost-containment in the social security system, and as a more-efficient response to the increase in demand for LTC services (Ikegami and Campbell, 2002; Villalobos Dintrans, 2018). Cost is usually the main argument against the implementation of an LTC system: the decision involves "extra" spending that is always hard for governments to assume. However, the right approach is to look at the benefits of the policy, not just the costs. The emphasis on reducing spending, mainly on health, together with the medicalization of care2 and the traditional view of LTC services as provided by families has contributed to the slow introduction of LTC systems around the world (Brodsky and Clarfield, 2008; European Union, 2016). The economic impact of an LTC system can be broadly analyzed from two perspectives (Villalobos Dintrans, 2018): i) effects on the labor market, as it can enhance dependents' and caregivers' participation in the formal labor market, and; ii) effects on public expenditures, as it increases the efficiency of the allocation and use of resources by offering cost-effective alternatives to respond to population needs (Rodrigues et al., 2013; Bloom et al., 2015; Rhee et al., 2015; World Health Organization, 2015; Norton, 2016).

[2] Medicalization is a process through which some aspects of human life come to be considered as medical problems, whereas before they were not considered as pathological. It can be defined as conceptual (when the medical lexicon is used to define non-medical entities), or interactional (when the physician, in interaction with the patient, redefines a social problem as a medical one) (Maturo, 2012).

Several studies using these perspectives have shown the huge financial impact of LTC when considering both the direct and indirect impacts, including the loss of productivity from informal caregiving (Arno et al., 1999; Rodrigues et al., 2013; Łyszczarz, 2019); the fostering of economic activity through creation of new markets (Choi, 2015; Jeon and Kwon, 2017); and general savings for the social security system (Campbell and Ikegami, 2000; Rhee et al., 2015; Norton, 2016; Villalobos Dintrans, 2018).

From a moral perspective, establishing LTC systems can help by dealing with a sense of unfairness in the society. Unfairness can be seen from different angles. On one hand, an LTC system provides a mechanism that facilitates intergenerational solidarity and clarifies the government's social responsibility. In this case, an LTC system helps by providing a public policy response to the otherwise default alternative: poor quality, unregulated services and intolerable burdens on caregivers and families (Ikegami and Campbell, 2002; Villalobos Dintrans 2018; 2019b; 2020). On the other hand, a public, comprehensive and universal system can help to satisfy people's desires to "share something equally" (Fuchs, 2011). This egalitarian feeling could be particularly relevant in countries with a fragmented social security system. First, though there could be disagreement on equality as a goal itself, the doctrine of egalitarianism has a counterpart in the doctrine of sufficiency: from a moral point of view, it is not important that everyone has the same, but it is morally important that each one has enough (Frankfurt, 2015). This is crucial in the debate on LTC and LTC systems and, as discussed, provides rationale for both the implementation of a system (versus the lack of one) and the establishment of a universal (national) system (versus the alternative of targeted services).

Second, the debate about the moral nature of inequality usually refers to wealth or income inequality. Even if we accept that income inequality is not morally wrong, we might not feel the same about other kinds of inequalities. Quoting Harry Frankfurt: "Insofar as economic inequality is undesirable, however, it is not because it is as such morally objectionable…To the extent that it truly is undesirable, it is on account of its almost irresistible tendency to generate unacceptable inequalities of other kinds" (2015, pp. x). We tend to tolerate more income inequality than, for example, health inequalities. The rationale for this specific egalitarianism relies on the premise that health is a special good because it is directly constitutive of a person's well-being and it enables the person to function as an agent3 (Anand, 2004; Daniels, 2007). The same idea is embedded in the concept of LTC. Similarly, Amartya Sen's capability approach, where a fair distribution of human capabilities is key to achieve social justice, also highlights the role of health (including functional ability) as a generator and barrier of opportunities and freedom to achieve (Sen, 1992; 2004). These ideas are embedded in the definition of LTC, and they highlight the need to consider both dependents and caregivers when thinking about LTC policies (World Health Organization, 2015). Thus, an LTC system is morally justified as an instrument to provide basic LTC services to those who need it (sufficiency) and to reduce differences in a dimension where equality is morally desirable.

Politically, LTC can also be viewed as a strategy. For example, Campbell et al. (2009) show how the introduction of LTC systems in Germany and Japan can be seen from a political perspective; responsiveness of the government to an evident and increasing problem can in fact attract voters (Campbell, 2002). The authors show how Japan's Golden Plan went from a campaign promise to become the cornerstone of the country's LTC system within years. Policies oriented toward older people can become more interesting for politicians because they help solve evident and urgent problems and because the pool of voters is aging.

Finally, countries have legal obligations towards their population. Many countries have established specific legal bodies to address this issue, particularly relating to LTC. Countries like the Netherlands, the Republic of Korea, Japan, France, Uruguay, and Germany have issued LTC-specific laws as part of the process of establishing their LTC systems. Other countries have broader regulations—mostly targeted at protecting people with disabilities or older people—that overlap with LTC initiatives, such as China, South Africa, Chile, or Indonesia; many include explicit mention of

---

[3] To pursue the various goals and projects in life that she has reason to value (Anand, 2004).

providing services to people in need of care in their constitutions (for example, Finland, Ethiopia, and South Africa). LTC-related legislation can be found in multiple places, whether explicitly addressing the issue of LTC, or as part of broader legislation pointing at health, social services, or special populations in need. Similarly, many countries have signed international treaties and agreements committing States to providing solutions to people with LTC needs.

4. Current and Future Challenges in Long-Term Care

The demographic and epidemiological changes, as well as the new perspectives regarding social security, present several challenges for countries around the world. Whether countries have made advances in implementing LTC systems or they are starting the debate around this topic, many unsolved issues are still pending. Moreover, the changing global and local context—including unexpected shocks such as the COVID-19 pandemic or political and social crises at the national level—imply extra efforts are needed for the task of providing LTC services and responding to people's needs.

4.1. Challenge 1: Establishing LTC Systems. Why is It Important for Developing Countries?

From a global perspective, one of the main issues regarding LTC is the immense number of countries in which LTC is still missing. As stated above, the WHO has made a call for the implementation of LTC systems in every country as a fundamental strategy for achieving healthy aging (World Health Organization, 2016; 2020a).

As explained above, despite common belief, LTC is not a "rich countries' problem". Developing countries will experience large and rapid increases in the demand for these services in the coming years. Unlike developed countries, developing countries have the opportunity to learn from the success and failures experienced by other nations in the implementation of their LTC systems. Unfortunately, given the speed of the coming changes, they will have less time to react. The particularities of the process of population aging confer on this policy (implementing a national LTC system) both a sense of relevance and urgency.

How can countries face this challenge? Following Kingdon's agenda-setting model (Kingdon, 1995), three elements are required to put a topic on the agenda and move from ideas into action: problem, policy, and politics.

To this end, countries should make efforts to improve their demographic data, in order to better describe the problem and work on feasible solutions. A first step requires understanding the country's situation in terms of LTC needs. For this, countries need to:

(i) set a definition of their LTC needs; and
(ii) collect data to estimate the demand for LTC services.

A detailed identification of the population's needs will help in designing solutions and defining the elements of an LTC system (Villalobos Dintrans, 2020). With this information, it is possible to make the case for an LTC system using, for example, some of the approaches described above (ethical, economic, political, legal). Involving public opinion as well as policy makers is key to moving forward on reforms to implement an LTC system.

4.2. Challenge 2: Improving LTC Systems. New Perspectives for LTC Systems Currently in Place

Although countries with an LTC system in place have already traveled part of the way, they still face several challenges to meet their population's needs. Several countries have been dealing with the implementation of their LTC systems for many years. These paths have demonstrated both lessons to learn and room for improvement. Some of the issues that are still being debated are related to financing, assessment of LTC needs, and quality. The issue of how to implement an LTC system that is sustainable, fair, and responsive to the people's needs is the topic of ongoing debate (Ikegami and Campbell, 2002; Swartz, 2013; Norton, 2016).

Financing is one of the most-discussed topics around LTC (Ikegami and Campbell, 2002; Brown and Finkelstein, 2009; Costa-Font and Courbage, 2012; Costa-Font et al., 2017). Countries are struggling with, on the one hand, implementing a financially sustainable LTC system and, on the other hand, providing more and better services for an increasing share of the population with LTC needs. There is no silver bullet for this problem, but countries have adopted different schemes—such as LTC social health insurance, tax-based systems, private insurance—in which families, the government, and the private sector contribute to finance LTC services. New financing schemes and more debate are expected in the coming years, particularly around the financing of LTC systems in more resource-constrained environments.

The discussion of LTC financing has minimized other issues that are relevant in the design and implementation of LTC systems (Villalobos Dintrans, 2020). One of the main issues of the LTC systems is the way in which they identify and select their beneficiaries. Countries have used the concept of dependency (functional, care) to operationalize the measurement and identification of LTC needs.

The lack of a consensus definition for LTC needs has pushed countries to adopt national definitions. Many of them have changed their definitions in recent years in order to include traditionally neglected populations for which the usual assessment instruments—based on the need for help performing activities of daily living (ADL)—cannot be used to identify LTC needs. In this group, for example, are children and people with mental health problems, particularly people with dementia. Countries like Germany and the Republic of Korea have recently changed their LTC assessment process to consider these populations (Federal Ministry of Health, 2009; Jeon and Kwon, 2017). These changes show the importance of reevaluating the concept of LTC needs and the tools available to assess it.

Finally, another never-ending discussion involves the quality of LTC services. Countries face a continual challenge regarding the quality of LTC services provided. Quality has been an issue, particularly linked to institutional care (Castle and Ferguson, 2010; Centers for Medicare & Medicaid Services, 2020). However, new trends in ways of providing LTC services, such as home-based LTC, and the idiosyncratic elements of each system (e.g., whether the system is universal or targeted, the public/ private nature of providers, the type of beneficiaries and benefits) pose different quality-related challenges (Brodsky and Clarfield, 2008; Villalobos Dintrans, 2020).

4.3. Challenge 3: The New World and LTC after COVID-19

The COVID-19 pandemic has changed the world. Many of the issues previously discussed will be impacted by this unexpected crisis. Although the relevance of LTC and LTC systems became even more relevant after the crisis, countries are expected to find additional challenges derived from the pandemic.

First, as LTC systems require funding, money is expected to be an issue, particularly because countries will prioritize resources for other areas of the health system, as well as for the reactivation of the economy. Mobilizing adequate funding for LTC to respond to and recover from the COVID-19 pandemic is identified as a key policy objective for countries (World Health Organization, 2020b).

On the other hand, health systems should also accommodate this new reality. Resource prioritization will not be the only relevant consideration in the post COVID-19 era; the role of health systems, particularly regarding LTC needs, will also be vital. The pandemic hit older people particularly hard, especially people living in LTC facilities. In every country, an important fraction of COVID-19 deaths was in older people (Ioannidis et al., 2020; Centers for Disease Control and Prevention, 2020).

Several countries reported that a large proportion of the deaths came from people living in LTC facilities (Comas-Herrera et al., 2020). Besides mortality issues, the pandemic also affected healthcare services overall (World Health Organization, 2020c). Measures to prevent spreading of the virus in the population—including lock downs and quarantines—were applied extensively. These measures can also have negative impacts on people's mental and physical health. These events are expected to have effects on people's functional abilities, increasing LTC needs in the population.

5. How to Move Forward?

Several challenges have been identified regarding the future of LTC around the world. The demographic and epidemiological transitions will pose pressure on countries in terms of provision of LTC services in the short term. These urgent needs, as well as other arguments to justify the implementation of LTC systems, should be seriously debated in every country.

The implementation of LTC systems is a complex issue, but an efficient LTC strategy is vital. Countries where there are currently no LTC institutions should start generating information to identify and measure the scale of the problem, as well as looking at the experiences of other countries to identify solutions.

For countries with LTC systems in place, several challenges are still pending: providing more and better services while ensuring the systems' sustainability is a never-ending problem. Fragmentation of services and silo financing of LTC initiatives are typical threats to improving LTC systems. Aligning the LTC system as part of the social security apparatus is a strategy that could help these countries move forward.

It is key for every country to act and highlight the relevance of LTC today. There is no time for waiting. Aged countries are already dealing with their LTC initiatives and "younger" countries will experience the increase in demand for these services soon. Delaying action on LTC means losing the valuable and scarce time that some countries might still have. Designing and implementing an LTC system is a long-term initiative, and acting now is necessary for countries to provide a response to their people in time.

This chapter has shown the importance of LTC today and for the coming years. Working together in the search for new solutions and the implementation of LTC systems around the world is a difficult but necessary step. Countries need to act today to respond to their people's needs.

References

Anand, S. (2004). The Concern for Equity in Health. In: Anand, S., Peter, F. and Sen, A. (Eds.). *Public Health, Ethics, and Equity*. Oxford: Oxford University Press.

Arno, P. S., Levine, C. & Memmott, M. M. (1999). The economic value of informal caregiving. *Health Affairs*, *18*, 182-188.

Bloom, D. E., Chatterji, S., Kowal, P., Lloyd-Sherlock, P., Mckee, M., Rechel, B., Rosenberg, L. & Smith, J. P. (2015). Macroeconomic implications of population ageing and selected policy responses. *Lancet*, *385*, 649-657.

Bongaarts, J. (2009). Human population growth and the demographic transition. *Philosophical Transactions of the Royal Society of London, Series B, Biological Sciences*, *364*(1532), 2985-2990.

Boutayeb, A. (2006). The double burden of communicable and non-communicable diseases in developing countries. *Transactions of The Royal Society of Tropical Medicine and Hygiene*, *100*(3), 191-199.

Brodsky, J. & Clarfield, A. M. (2008). Long term care in health services. In: Heggenhougen, H. K. and Quah, S. (Eds.). *International Encyclopedia of Public Health*. San Diego: Academic Press.

Brown, J. R. & Finkelstein, A. (2009). The private market for long-term care insurance in the U.S.: A review of the evidence. *Journal of Risk and Insurance*, *76*(1), 5-29.

Bygbjerg, I. C. (2012). Double Burden of Noncommunicable and Infectious Diseases in Developing Countries. *Science*, *337*(6101), 1499-1501.

Campbell, J. C. (2002). How policies differ: Long-term care insurance in Japan and Germany. In: Conrad, H. and Lützeler, R. (Eds.). *Aging and social policy - A German-Japanese comparison*. Munich; Iudicium.

Campbell, J. C. & Ikegami, N. (2000). Long-term care insurance comes to Japan. *Health Affairs*, *19*, 26-39.

Campbell, J. C., Ikegami, N. & Kwon, S. (2009). Policy learning and cross-national diffusion in social long-term care insurance: Germany, Japan, and the Republic of Korea. *International Social Security Review*, *62*(4), 63-80.

Carrera, F., Pavolini, E., Ranci, C. & Sabbatini, A. (2013). Long-term care systems in comparative perspective: Care needs, informal and formal coverage, and social impacts in European countries. In: Ranci, C. and Pavolini, F. (Eds.). *Reforms in long-term care policies in Europe*. New York: Springer.

Castle, N. G. & Ferguson, J. C. (2010). What is nursing home quality and how is it measured? *The Gerontologist*, *50*(4), 426-442.

Centers for Disease Control and Prevention. (2020). *Weekly Updates by Select Demographic and Geographic Characteristics*. Available from: https://www.cdc.gov/nchs/nvss/vsrr/covid_weekly/index.htm [4 Sep 2020].

Centers for Medicare & Medicaid Services. (2020). *Ensuring safety and quality in America's nursing homes.* Available from: https://www.cms.gov/blog/ensuring-safety-and-quality-americas-nursing-homes [29 Aug 2020].

Choi, Y. J. (2015). *Long-Term Care of Older Persons in the Republic of Korea. SDD-SPPS Project Working Papers Series: Long-Term Care for Older Persons in Asia and the Pacific*. Available from: https://www.unescap.org/sites/default/files/Long-term%20care%20for%20older%20persons%20in%20the%20Republic%20of%20Korea.pdf [29 Jul 2020].

Colombo, C., Llena-Nozal, A., Mercier, J. & Tjadens, F. (2011). *Help Wanted. Providing and Paying for Long-Term Care*. Paris: OECD Publishing.

Comas-Herrera, A., Zalakaín, J., Litwin, C., Hsu, A. T., Lemmon, E., Henderson, D. & Fernández, J. L. (2020). *Mortality associated with COVID-19 outbreaks in care homes: early international evidence. International Long-Term Care Policy Network, CPEC-LSE*. Available at: https://ltccovid.org/wp-content/uploads/2020/06/Mortality-associated-with-COVID-among-people-who-use-long-term-care-26-June-1.pdf [4 Sep 2020].

Costa-Font, J. & Courbage, C (Eds.). (2012). *Financing long-term care in Europe. Institutions, markets and models*. Basingstoke, UK: Palgrave Macmillan.

Costa-Font, J., Courbage, C. & Zweifel, P. (2017). Policy dilemmas in financing long-term care in Europe. *Global Policy*, *8*(2), 38-45.

Daniels, N. (2007). *Just Health: Meeting Health Needs Fairly*. Cambridge: Cambridge University Press.

European Union. (2016). *Joint report on health care and long-term care systems and fiscal sustainability.* Institutional Paper 037. European Commission.

Federal Ministry of Health. (2009) *Report by the advisory board to review the definition of the need for long-term care*. Available from: https://www.bundesgesundheitsministerium.de/fileadmin/Dateien/3_Downloads/E/Englische_Dateien/Report_by_the_advisory_board_to_review_the_definition_of_the_need_for_long-term_care.pdf [29 Aug 2020].

Freedman, V. A., Martin, L. G., Cornman, J., Agree, E. M. & Schoeni, R. F. (2008). Trends in Assistance with Daily Activities: Racial/ Ethnic and Socioeconomic Disparities Persist in the U. S. Older Population. In: Cutler, D. M. and Wise, D. A. (Eds.). *Health at Older Ages: The Causes and Consequences of Declining Disability among the Elderly*. Chicago: University of Chicago Press.

Frankfurt, H. G. (2015). *On inequality*. Princeton: Princeton University Press.

Fuchs, V. R. (1999). “Provide, Provide”: The Economics of Aging. In: Rettermair, A. J. and Savings, T. R. (Eds.). *Medicare Reform: Issues and Answers*. Chicago: University of Chicago Press.

Fuchs, V. R. (2011). *Who Shall Live? Health, Economics and Social Choice. 2nd Expanded Edition*. New Jersey: World Scientific.

Geraedts, M., Heller, G. V. & Harrington, C. A. (2000). Germany’s long-term-care insurance: putting a social insurance model into practice. *Milbank Quarterly*, *78*, 375-401.

Ikegami, N. & Campbell, J. C. (2002). Choices, Policy Logics and Problems in the Design of Long-Term Care Systems. *Social Policy & Administration*, *36*(7), 719-734.

Institute for Health Metrics and Evaluation (2017). *GBD Compare* | Viz Hub. Retrieved from: https://vizhub.healthdata.org/gbd-compare/ [21 Jul 2020].

Institute for Health Metrics and Evaluation (2020). *Frequently Asked Questions*. Retrieved from: http://www.healthdata.org/gbd/ FAQ# What%20is%20a%20DALY? [25 Jul 2020].

Ioannidis, J. P. A., Axfors, C. & Contopoulos-Ioannidis, D. G. (2020). Population-level COVID-19 mortality risk for non-elderly individuals overall and for non-elderly individuals without underlying diseases in pandemic epicenters. *Environmental Research*, *188*, 109890.

Jeon, B. & Kwon, S. (2017). Health and long-term care systems for older people in the Republic of Korea: policy challenges and lessons. *Health Systems & Reform*, *3*, 214-223.

Kingdon, J. W. (1995). *Agendas, Alternatives, and Public Policies. Second Edition*. New York: HarperCollins.

Lee, R. (2003). The Demographic Transition: Three Centuries of Fundamental Change. *Journal of Economic Perspectives*, *17*(4), 167–190.

Lee, R. (2011). The Outlook for Population Growth. *Science*, *333*(6042), 569-573.

Łyszczarz, B. (2019). Indirect costs and incidence of caregivers’ short-term absenteeism in Poland, 2006–2016. *BMC Public Health*, *19*, 598.

Malthus, T. R. (1798/1993). *An Essay on the Principle of Population*. Oxford: Oxford University Press.

Manton, K. G. & Stallard, E. (1994). Medical Demography: Interaction of Disability Dynamics and Mortality. In: Martin, L. G. and Preston, S. H. (Eds.). *Demography of Aging*. Washington: National Academy Press.

Maturo, A. (2012). Medicalization: Current Concept and Future Directions in a Bionic Society. *Mens Sana Monographs*, *10*(1), 122-133.

McKeown, R. E. (2009). The Epidemiologic Transition: Changing Patterns of Mortality and Population Dynamics. *American Journal of Lifestyle Medicine*, *3*(1 Suppl), 19S-26S.

Mot, E. (2010). *The long-term care system for the elderly in the Netherlands.* ENEPRI research report 90, European Network of Economic Policy Research Institutes.

Norton, E. C. (2016). Health and Long-Term Care. In: Piggott, J. and Woodland, A. (Eds.). *Handbook of the Economics of Population Aging*, Volume *1B*. Amsterdam: North-Holland.

Omran, A. R. (1971). The Epidemiologic Transition: A Theory of the Epidemiology of Population Change. *Milbank Memorial Fund Quarterly*, *49*(4, Part 1), 509-538.

Rhee, J. C., Done, N. & Anderson, G. F. (2015). Considering long-term care insurance for middle-income countries: comparing South Korea with Japan and Germany. *Health Policy*, *119*, 1319-1329.

Rodrigues, R., Schulmann, K., Schmidt, A., Kalavrezou, N. & Matsaganis, M. (2013). The indirect costs of long-term care. Research note 8/2013, European Commission.

Sen, A. (1992). *Inequality reexamined.* Cambridge: Harvard University Press.

Sen, A. (2004). Why Health Equity?. In: Anand, S., Peter, F. and Sen, A. (Eds.). *Public Health, Ethics, and Equity*. Oxford: Oxford University Press.

Swartz, K. (2013). Searching for a Balance of Responsibilities: OECD Countries' Changing Elderly Assistance Policies. *Annual Review of Public Health*, 34, 397-412.

United Nations. (n.d.). *Dependency ratio*. Retrieved from: https://www.un.org/esa/sustdev/natlinfo/indicators/methodology_sheets/demographics/dependency_ratio.pdf [20 Jul 2020].

United Nations. (2019). *World Population Prospects 2019*. Retrieved from: https://population.un.org/wpp/ [20 Jul 2020].

Villalobos Dintrans, P. (2018). Long-term care systems as social security: the case of Chile. *Health Policy and Planning*, *33*(9), 1018-1025.

Villalobos Dintrans, P. (2019a). Long-term care in Chile: The faces of dependency. *ReVista: Harvard Review of Latin America*. Winter 2019 (Aging in the Americas). Retrieved from: https:// revista.drclas.harvard.edu/book/long-term-care-chile [20 Jul 2020].

Villalobos Dintrans, P. (2019b). Informal caregivers in Chile: the equity dimension of an invisible burden. *Health Policy and Planning*, *34*(10), 792-799.

Villalobos Dintrans, P. (2020). Designing Long-Term Care Systems: Elements to Consider. *Journal of Aging & Social Policy*, *32*(1), 83-99.

World Health Organization. (1999). *The World Health Report: Making a Difference*. Geneva: World Health Organization.

World Health Organization. (2015). *World Report on Ageing and Health*. Geneva: World Health Organization.

World Health Organization. (2016). *Global Strategy and Action Plan on Ageing and Health: A Framework for Coordinated Global Action by the World Health Organization, Member States, and Partners across the Sustainable Development Goals*. Geneva: World Health Organization.

World Health Organization. (2020a). *Decade of Healthy Ageing 2020-2030*. Geneva: World Health Organization.

World Health Organization. (2020b). *Preventing and managing COVID-19 across long-term care services. Policy brief.* Geneva: World Health Organization.

World Health Organization. (2020c). *Pulse survey on continuity of essential health services during the COVID-19 pandemic: interim report, 27 August 2020.* Geneva: World Health Organization.

In: The Future of Long-Term Care
Editor: Pablo Villalobos Dintrans
ISBN: 978-1-53619-263-6

Chapter 2

THE FUTURE OF LONG-TERM CARE IN DEVELOPING COUNTRIES: INSIGHTS FROM TURKEY

***Fatih Cemil Ozbugday*[1,*] *and Abdullah Tirgil*[2]**
[1]Department of Economics, Ankara Yıldırım Beyazıt University, Ankara, Turkey
[2]Department of Public Finance, Ankara Yıldırım Beyazıt University, Ankara, Turkey

ABSTRACT

The economic research on long-term care (LTC) has mostly focused on developed countries with high income per capita. Even though these countries' economic, demographic, and cultural characteristics are not exactly the same, a common topic of the research in developed countries is that demand and supply factors of LTC will put significant pressures on the sustainability of public finances. In other words, the future financial sustainability of LTC is in jeopardy for many developed countries. While economic research on LTC in developing countries is scarce, the same conclusions are not necessarily applicable in this setting. The economic, demographic, and cultural characteristics that affect the

* Corresponding Author's E-mail: fcbugday@gmail.com.

demand for and supply of LTC services are likely to be very different in developing countries compared with developed ones. This study focuses on how these characteristics influence the demand for and supply of LTC in Turkey, a developing country. We first provide an overview of the institutional background of LTC delivery in Turkey. We then discuss what LTC's future might look like in Turkey and compare this with developed countries.

1. INTRODUCTION

Colombo et al. (2011) define long-term care (LTC) as

> "a range of services required by persons with a reduced degree of functional capacity, physical or cognitive, and who are consequently dependent for an extended period of time on help with basic activities of daily living (ADL)." (Colombo et al., 2011)

Even though there is no age dimension in this definition, the primary recipients of LTC are older people. LTC can be offered either as *residential care* in nursing homes or as *home-based care* at the home of the individual who needs LTC. Residential care is usually formal care provided by paid and professionally trained workers, while home-based care can be provided either formally by paid professionals or informally by family members or relatives.

There is plentiful research on LTC in subfields of economic literature such as health economics, public economics, labor economics, industrial organization, and household economics (Ozbugday et al., 2020). The research on LTC is concerned with a wide range of subjects, including but not limited to: the optimal organization of LTC services delivery (Kim and Norton, 2017; Gaughan et al., 2017); the financing model of LTC to restrain public LTC spending (Costa-Font and Patxot, 2004; Fukui and Iwamoto, 2007; Costa-Font et al., 2015; Wouterse and Smid, 2017); the connection between LTC and healthcare (Yang et al., 2003); analyses of informal care provision (Pezzin et al., 1996; Charles and Sevak, 2005; Bolin et al., 2008; Bonsang, 2009); the impact of regulation and competition on quality of LTC service provision (Bowlbis et al., 2012;

Forder and Allan, 2014); the design of LTC insurance (Courbage and Eeckhoudt, 2012); and government subsidies to LTC (Kim and Lim, 2015). All these articles, as well as many others not cited here, use data and samples from developed countries such as the United States, Japan, the Netherlands, South Korea, and the United Kingdom, among others. Thus, economic research on LTC has mostly focused on developed countries with high income per capita. The primary reason for the dominance of developed countries in LTC research is that the aggregate demand for LTC is high in these countries because of their socio-demographic characteristics. For example, with the aging of the population, the very old-age dependency ratio—the share of people aged 80+ per 100 people of working age—has increased in these countries, which, in turn, has boosted the demand for LTC. Another socio-demographic characteristic of developed countries related to LTC demand is aggregate income. These developed countries are mostly welfare states that could afford public financing of formal LTC. Finally, cultural factors such as attitudes towards elderly family members could be other determinants of LTC arrangement decisions (Costa-Font, 2010; Gentili et al., 2017).

Another reason for the abundance of studies on LTC in developed countries is the availability and quality of data. Developed countries collect a series of data ranging from the quality ratings of nursing homes to individual characteristics of LTC recipients, which allows for a rich literature on LTC, to which many scholars contribute empirical analyses, to flourish.

Even though the economic, demographic, and cultural characteristics of developed countries are not exactly the same, a common theme of the research on LTC in developed countries is that demand and supply factors of LTC will put significant pressures on the long-term sustainability of public financing of LTC in these economies (Ozbugday et al., 2020). A relevant question, then, is what is the current situation and what will happen to LTC in developing economies? Do they share the same destiny as developed countries, or does a different future await them? Even though we may not know the answers to these questions with certainty, comparing the current situation and future projections in developing economies to those of developed economies can provide an idea of what we should expect.

The story of LTC could be different for developing economies due to their unique economic, demographic, and cultural characteristics. For example, if the very-old age dependency ratio is low in a developing country because of its population structure, then the demand for LTC will be significantly less (even if the population aging process will happen faster in such a country). Alternatively, if a society's cultural features require that the older people who need assistance should be given care by their family members or relatives, then the demand for formal LTC by professional paid workers will be reduced. Furthermore, if the prevalence of dementia in a developing country (a critical factor for aggregate LTC demand) is high, then we can expect more reliance on LTC for the older people there.

This chapter focuses on Turkey, a developing country, and contributes to the scarce literature on LTC provision in developing countries. The related literature mostly revolves around studies on developed economies, with just a few exceptions studying developing countries (Hirschfeld and Hirschfeld, 2003; Villalobos Dintrans, 2018, 2019a, 2019b). More generally, we focus on how economic, demographic, and cultural factors can influence the demand and supply of LTC in Turkey.

This chapter is organized as follows: Section 2 presents an overview of Turkey's LTC system, providing the institutional background of LTC delivery in Turkey. Section 3 displays the projections of factors that could affect the demand and supply of LTC in Turkey for the future, in order to provide a comparison with developed countries. Finally, Section 4 discusses these findings and draws conclusions from them.

2. An Overview of Turkey's Long-Term Care System

Turkey is an upper-middle-income country located in Europe and Central Asia, with a population of 83.15 million in 2019. Turkey's GDP per capita increased from USD 509 in 1960 to USD 9,042 in 2019. The proportion of total health expenditure to gross domestic product (%) was 4.4% in 2018 (TurkStat).

Turkey differs from other countries in terms of its demographic characteristics. The distribution of the population by age groups in 2019 was: 23.1% of children aged 0-14, 67.8% of adults aged 15-64, and 9.1% of older people aged 65 or over. Life expectancy at birth in Turkey increased significantly from 70 years in 2000 to 77 years in 2018. Moreover, the total fertility rate (births per woman) in Turkey declined from 3.1 in 1990 to 2.1 in 2018 (TurkStat, 2020).

The number of older people aged 80 and above in 2013 was 1,261,273. This number went up to 1,315,845 in 2014, and in 2015 increased to 1,328,924. Also, the number of older people aged 90 and above was 89,709 in 2012, and this number increased to 99,005 in 2013, 115,277 in 2014, and 127,986 in 2015. It is important to note here that the percent increase in the number of older people aged 90+ from 2012 to 2013 was 10%, 16% from 2013 to 2014, and 11% from 2014 to 2015. Furthermore, Özmete and Hussein (2017) reported that the leading causes of death for adults in Turkey in 2014 were diseases of the circulatory system (46.7%), malignant neoplasms (16.9%), and respiratory system diseases (12.8%). Alzheimer's disease is one of the diseases that require long-term care. In Turkey in 2014, the proportion of adults who died from Alzheimer's was 4%, up from 2.7% in 2010. This outcome may indicate that there will be an increase in demand for LTC services due to Alzheimer's disease going forward.

Considering these demographic and epidemiologic transitions, Turkey has been providing services for people with disabilities and older people since the early 1980s under Social Services Law No. 2828. Institutional care has been the primary method for helping functionally, socially, and economically deprived older people in Turkey. Nursing homes and care and rehabilitation centers were established across the country over time. Then, Disability Law No. 5378 provided an opportunity for home-based LTC services in 2005, which allowed older people and people with disabilities to obtain LTC services without leaving their social and physical environment.

Since 2005, with the modification of the Disability Law, the Ministry of Family and Social Policy (MFSP), now Ministry of Family, Labor and Social Services, has been in charge of the standardization, development, and dissemination of support and care services, while the Ministry of National Education (MoE) conducts the services related to special education for people with disabilities. For this reason, daycare centers providing special education and rehabilitation services were closed. Centers that continue to serve this population were changed to include mainly group work and to provide half or full day care services.

Provision of LTC for older people in Turkey increased its pace in the mid-2000s. For example, in 2007, a National Action Plan was introduced to deal with the situation of older people and general population aging, in which actions were planned to address access to health care and LTC, support the mental health of older people, and educate those who offer LTC (Özmete and Hussein, 2017). In 2011, Turkey established the MFSP, which determines which people with disabilities and older people are in need, and implements the required services for their protection, care, and rehabilitation. The MFSP also establishes and operates day and residential care institutions to provide LTC services. The General Directorate of People with Disability and Older People Services (GDDES) of the MFSP is responsible for establishing the necessary tools to provide social support to these people, as well as standardizing, monitoring and inspecting existing services (Ayhan, 2014). In addition to this, municipalities, charitable foundations, private institutions, and similar organizations also offer LTC services in Turkey.

For the first time, within the scope of its 10th development plan (2014-2018), the Ministry of Development created a specialized commission on aging in July 2013. In this plan, Turkey identified strategies for aging and LTC services. The GDDES started to work on care assurance models and care insurance within the scope of the Care Services Strategies and Action Plan (2011-2013), which focused on why Turkey needed to introduce LTC insurance and how to finance it.

Furthermore, in 2015, the Ministry of Health (MoH) introduced Turkey's Healthy Aging Action Plan and Application Program (2015-2020), where they based their work on four significant concepts: i) Lifelong Health Promotion and Healthy Aging; ii) Protection of Society from Health Risks; iii) Development of Health Services for Older People and Health Services Ensuring Full Access, and; iv) Strengthening Monitoring and Evaluation. In the meantime, the GDDES carried out a pilot of an Active Aging Strategy with several participating institutions, such as universities, municipalities, related public institutions, and non-governmental institutions.

To assist municipalities in providing care services for older people, the MFSP introduced the older people support program (YADES), which covers people aged 65 and older. YADES provides protection and support for older people and aims to provide some care in their home environment. For this purpose, the MFSP provides resources and budget to municipalities. Figure 1 displays a timeline showing the main milestones regarding LTC in Turkey.

Today, the primary provider of LTC services in Turkey is the Ministry of Family, Labor and Social Services (MFLSS), previously known as the MFSP. Municipalities, charitable foundations, and others can also offer these services to some extent. The MFLSS is responsible for identifying people with disabilities and older people who need LTC and establishing places where they can obtain the services they need. The MFLSS is also responsible for checking private and other institutions that offer LTC services to ensure they provide standardized and high-quality care.

The main message that the MFLSS conveys is the importance of providing LTC services to people with disabilities and older people at home, without separating them from their families. Under Law No. 6518, it states that

> "necessary psychosocial support and care services are provided in accordance with the situation so that people with disability can live independently in their environment. In the provision of support and care services, the biological, physical, psychological, social, cultural, and spiritual needs of the person are considered, by considering their family."

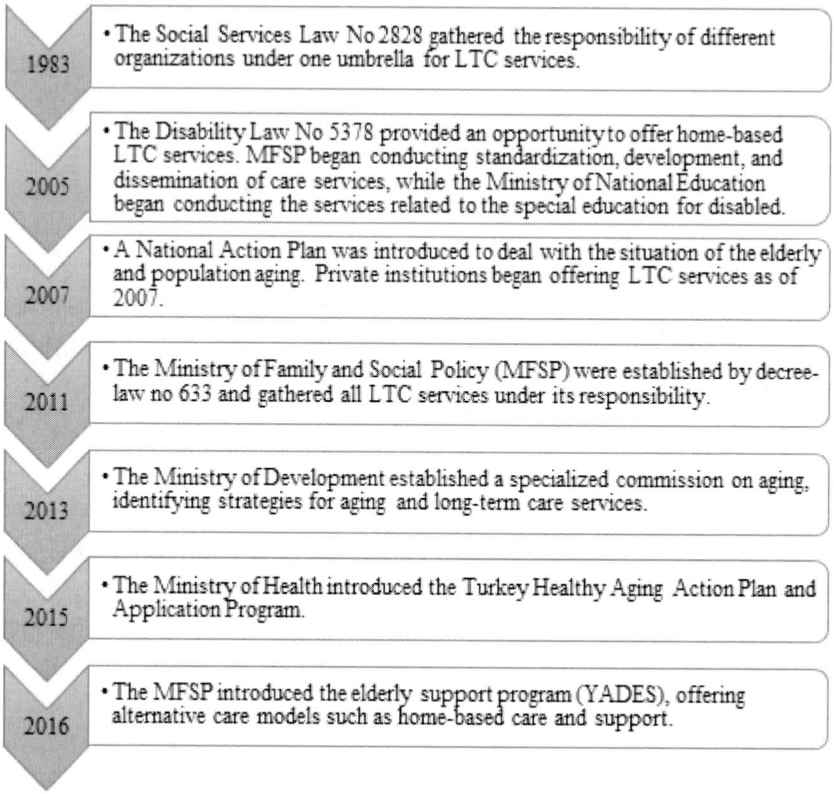

Figure 1. Main milestones regarding LTC in Turkey.

The authorities do everything in their power to achieve this purpose. However, if home-based care is not feasible, institutional LTC is offered at designated formal or private institutions.

The LTC system in Turkey comprises two principal systems, including the health and social sectors. The health component of the LTC system for older people is provided by the Chronic Diseases, Older People's Health, and Handicapped Department (CDOHHD) under the MoH, which focuses on developing national health programs concerning older people's health, prevention of disability, and carrying out home-based health services. The MoH in Turkey is responsible for offering LTC health services, including providing physicians and hospital care. Also, the MoH oversees the home-based health care services provided by physicians, nurses, and other health personnel across the country by visiting people with disabilities and older people in need in their home environment.

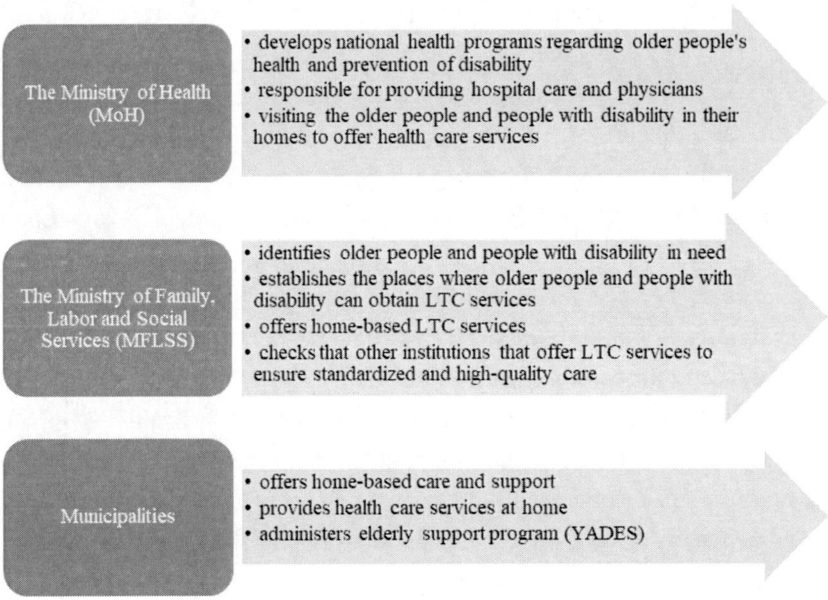

Figure 2. Institutional arrangements in LTC in Turkey.

Since the enactment of the Disability Law No. 5378, Turkey has changed its LTC services from an institutionalized structure to one focused on home-based and community-based LTC (see Figure 2). In 2006, only six (6) people were benefiting from home-based care, while in 2016 this number increased to 478,319. There is no LTC insurance in Turkey. Instead, Turkey finances LTC services through general budget revenues. To provide health care services to people with disabilities and older people in need of LTC, financing comes through the social security system provided by universal health coverage (Bal, 2016; Ağören, 2017).

In the next section, we will focus on the four components of LTC according to the framework developed by Villalobos Dintrans (2020): beneficiaries, benefit package, providers, and financing.

2.1. Beneficiaries of LTC in Turkey and Eligibility Criteria

For policymakers, defining the beneficiaries of LTC services is as important as its implementation. Turkey defines the LTC system's beneficiaries under Decree-Law No. 633, which established two types of beneficiaries of LTC services: people with disabilities and older people in need of care. According to the country's disability classification, people with disabilities in need of care is defined as a person who has been documented to be severely disabled by an official medical board report, and who is unable to continue his/her life without the help and care of someone else because of difficulties in carrying out activities of daily living (ADL). Obtaining medical board certification is not enough to certify the need for care. Afterward, the MFLSS province directorates must validate this certificate, investigating whether the person is having difficulties in carrying out ADL without the help of others. Based on the care report form, it is decided whether the person is indeed in need of care. An older person in need of care is defined as one who needs protection, care, and assistance.

Turkey offers LTC in different forms, such as home-based care, houses of hope, nursing homes, care and rehabilitation centers, and old life houses. For those who offer home-based care to people with disabilities, the government provides home-care allowances, to provide financial protection for caregivers and families. The home-care allowance aims at providing personal care and support to those in need who are being cared for by their relatives.

The home-care allowance depends on three critical conditions (Karakuş, 2018):

1) The person is severely disabled (50% or more) which can be verified through the medical board report (disability condition),
2) The person with disabilities cannot carry out ADL without the help and care of others, which must be validated by the MFLSS province directorates (functional dependency condition),

3) The monthly household income per person is less than two-thirds of the net minimum wage (mean-tested condition).

If the person with disabilities meets these three conditions, then he/she can obtain the home-care allowance. Caregivers also need to meet some requirements. First, the person with disabilities and the caregiver have to live in the same household or a close vicinity in order for caregivers to be able to offer 24-hour service in case of need. Although it is expected that the caregiver is typically a relative of the people with disabilities, non-relatives can also provide LTC. Finally, caregivers must provide LTC services for at least eight (8) hours a day (Karakuş, 2018; Özmete and Hussein, 2017).

As mentioned before, Turkey offers different LTC services for older people in need, including nursing homes, care and rehabilitation centers, and old life houses. Applicants must meet the conditions listed below in order to receive LTC services in public or private nursing homes (Özmete and Hussein, 2017):

1) Aged 60 or older,
2) Difficulty in carrying out ADL such as eating, bathing, going to the restroom, and dressing without the help and care of others,
3) Good mental health,
4) No contagious disease,
5) No drug or alcohol dependence,
6) A committee must certify social and economic deprivation.

To be able to benefit from older people and rehabilitation centers, applicants must meet the requirements below:

1. Aged 60 or older,
2. Need for special attention, support, and rehabilitation due to their physical and mental condition,
3. Mental health problems,
4. No contagious disease,
5. No drug or alcohol dependence,

6. Social services professionals in provinces check whether the residents meet these requirements.

2.2. LTC Services and LTC Providers in Turkey

Formal and informal care are the two ways of addressing dependents' LTC needs. Formal care is mostly received in nursing homes and care and rehabilitation centers. On the other hand, home-based care is mostly provided by family members or friends, usually in the form of informal care.

Like other countries—such as the Netherlands and the Republic of Korea—Turkey recently changed to provide more community-based LTC instead of institutional LTC services (Swartz, 2013). One of the reasons countries opt for home-based care is because formal care is more expensive, which may challenge countries' financial systems (Lipszyc et al., 2012), especially developing ones. Another likely explanation is that dependents prefer home-based care provided by their relatives or friends (Özmete and Hussein, 2017). According to Turkey's Family Structure Survey, when people aged 60 and below were asked where they think they would live when they get older, 22.7% of respondents responded "they would stay with their son"; 19.6% responded "they would stay home and receive home-based care"; 8.7% responded "they would stay with their daughters"; and 10.3% responded, "they would stay in nursing homes."

Turkey handles the cases of people with disabilities and older people in need of care separately. People with disabilities are offered institutional care through residential care centers, daycare, house of hope, private care centers, and home-based care. On the other hand, for older people in need of care, Turkey provides LTC through nursing homes, care and rehabilitation centers, private nursing homes, old life houses, and home-based care.

2.2.1. Home-Based Care

Home-based care offers individuals cleaning services, cooking, washing clothes, tooth brushing, personal care, and similar needs 24 hours a day (Özmete and Hussein, 2017). The purpose of offering home-based care services to people with disability in need is to allow them to stay in their social and physical environment.

Home-based care LTC services were introduced in 2006, and only eight (8) individuals benefited from these services at the time; this figure increased to 526,754 individuals in March 2020. Turkey does not allow professional caregivers to offer home-based LTC services. Besides services like cleaning, cooking, washing, and other services, the Ministry of Health (MoH) provides health care services to people with disabilities in their homes. It is important to note that those who benefit from home-based care services are evaluated based on their level of disability, not their age.

Table 1 shows the distribution of people with disabilities benefiting from home-care assistance and the payments made by the state budget every year (2007-2020). Table 1 reports that the number of people with disabilities benefiting from home-care allowances was 28,583 in 2007, which increased 18-fold by March 2020. It is important to note that about one-third of the people with disabilities benefited from the home-care allowance were also older people (Karakuş, 2018). The table shows how the number of people with disabilities benefiting from home-care support increases year by year, which also supports the importance of community-based LTC solutions in Turkey.

Besides, the MFSP (now MFLSS) introduced the YADES program in 2016, which provides financial support from the general budget to some municipalities, in order to offer LTC services to older people. YADES aims at providing daycare and home-based LTC to those aged 65 years and older without changing their environment, as an alternative to institutional care.

Table 1. Number of people with disabilities benefiting from home care assistance and the amount of payment by years

Year	Number of people with disabilities	Total payment (million USD)
2020 (March)	526,754	-
2019	514,158	1,527
2018	506,725	1,808
2017	499,130	1,647
2016	478,711	1,742
2015	464,741	1,609
2014	450,036	1,864
2013	425,928	1,992
2012	398,335	1,561
2011	347,756	1,424
2010	279,580	1,062
2009	204,652	627
2008	113,000	356
2007	28,583	24

Source: General Directorate of People with Disabilities and Older People Services (2020).

2.2.2. Institutional Care

Turkey has been experiencing social, economic, and cultural transformations for decades, in the form of migration from villages to cities, increased labor force participation by women (who are culturally considered to be the primary person responsible for LTC in the family), and transition from extended family to a nuclear family, all of which have led to an increase in the demand for institutional LTC. Furthermore, insufficient skills of family members, especially in situations that require health care interventions, have also increased the need for institutional care (Seyyar, 2013).

As stated before, people with disabilities and older people in need of care can benefit from institutional LTC in Turkey in different forms, such as nursing homes, care and rehabilitation centers, and day care centers. Since 2007, private institutions have been offering LTC services to meet the increased demand. Therefore, if people with disabilities cannot benefit from home-based care, it is possible to send them to private institutions to receive the required LTC services upon their family's request.

Table 2. Number of people with disabilities benefiting from residential and day care and associated capacities

Year	Total number of people living in residential care (1)	Total number of people receiving day care (2)	Total number of people receiving benefits (1) + (2)	Total capacit y
2020 (March)	7,064	790	7,854	8,293
2019	7,383	735	8,118	8,289
2018	7,305	440	7,745	7,869
2017	7,240	459	7,699	7,925
2016	7,096	411	7,507	7,458
2015	6,494	432	6,926	6,992
2014	5,827	457	6,284	6,682
2013	5,451	441	5,892	6,293
2012	5,112	460	5,586	6,055
2011	4,708	454	5,162	5,833
2010	4,490	415	4,905	5,468
2009	4,190	379	4,569	4,758
2008	3,802	470	4,272	4,098
2007	3,458	634	4,092	3,434
2006	3,070	1,584	4,654	3,027
2005	2,658	2,287	4,945	2,755
2004	2,441	1,978	4,419	2,415
2003	2,162	2,768	4,930	2,086
2002	1,843	2,065	3,908	1,943

Notes: Residential care includes care provided at rehabilitation centers and houses of hope.
Source: General Directorate of People with Disabilities and Older People Services (2020).

Table 2 shows the number of people with disabilities receiving official care, including residential care, rehabilitation centers, and daycare. While the number of people with disabilities receiving care was 1,843 in 2002, this number increased to 7,064 by March 2020. On the other hand, the number of people with disabilities who benefited from daycare was 2,065 in 2002. This number decreased to 790 by March 2020. The last column shows the capacities of these centers.

Table 3 shows the distribution of people with disabilities receiving care in private centers, and the resources allocated to this scheme. Private care centers for people with disabilities began providing LTC services in

2007 with only 10 care centers. This number went up to 267 as of March 2020, serving 19,931 people with disabilities.

Table 3. Distribution of people with disabilities receiving care services in private care centers and resources allocated

Year	Number of centers	Capacity	Number of people with disabilities receiving care	Total public expenditures (million USD)
2020 (March)	267	25,684	19,931	-
2019	257	24,796	19,658	144
2018	231	21,200	17,264	144
2017	196	17,690	14,080	112
2016	161	14,236	11,923	86
2015	156	13,656	10,823	94
2014	149	13,443	10,319	92
2013	147	13,325	10,173	104
2012	148	12,869	9,328	72
2011	100	8,651	6,707	54
2010	77	7,065	4,331	30
2009	44	3,744	2,144	11
2008	20	2,003	768	4
2007	10	915	351	0.69

Source: General Directorate of People with Disabilities and Older People Services (2020).

Table 4 reports the distribution of nursing homes affiliated with the MFLSS and the number of older people living in these centers (residents). The number of nursing homes increased 2.5 times between 2002 and 2020. However, the capacity of these centers was always greater than the number of older people staying in them except in 2011. We report more detailed statistics on columns 4-6. Column 4 reports the average capacity, which stayed almost the same between 2002 and March 2020. Column 5 shows the average occupancy for the same years, indicating a 15% increase. Finally, we also report the percent excess of capacity in column 6, where we observe a 13% decline in the excess capacity of nursing homes affiliated with the MFLSS between 2002 and 2020.

Table 4. Distribution of nursing homes affiliated to the MFLSS and number of older people staying in these centers

Years	Number of nursing homes (1)	Capacity (2)	Number of older people (residents) (3)	Average capacity (capacity/ number of nursing homes) (4)	Average occupancy (residents/ number of nursing homes) (5)	% excess of capacity ([capacity-residents]/ capacity) (6)
2020	153	15,649	13,868	102	91	0.11
2019	153	15,385	13,888	101	91	0.10
2018	146	14,967	13,883	103	95	0.07
2017	144	14,793	13,692	103	95	0.07
2016	141	14,412	13,248	102	94	0.08
2015	132	13,488	12,299	102	93	0.09
2014	124	12,647	11,688	102	94	0.08
2013	115	12,241	11,293	106	98	0.08
2012	106	11,706	10,951	110	103	0.06
2011	102	9,783	10,590	96	104	-0.08
2010	97	9,260	7,979	95	82	0.14
2009	81	8,126	7,220	100	89	0.11
2008	79	8,002	6,773	101	86	0.15
2007	70	7,552	6,477	108	93	0.14
2006	69	7,605	6,082	110	88	0.20
2005	66	7,173	5,603	109	85	0.22
2004	62	6,760	5,389	109	87	0.20
2003	63	6,580	5,188	104	82	0.21
2002	63	6,477	4,952	103	79	0.24

Source: General Directorate of People with Disability and Older People Services (2020). Year 2020 reports statistics until March.

2.2.3. Community-Based Care

Turkey tends to provide community-based LTC services to keep people with disabilities and older people in their home environments, which would enable their continued integration with the rest of society. Policymakers believe that offering LTC services in an environment where people feel at home will result in physically and mentally healthier individuals later in life (Ayhan, 2014). For this purpose, Turkey developed new practices within the framework of the community-based care model such as houses of hope and old life houses. For example, a "house of hope" has been established for people with disabilities to live in an environment with their neighbors, using an apartment or detached house. These houses are composed of twelve individuals. There are four bedrooms, each of which is shared by three people. The houses have a living room, kitchen, dining hall, toilet, bathroom, and staff room. They are detached single floor and garden houses.

Table 5 shows the distribution of residential care, including care and rehabilitation centers, and the houses of hope for the people with disabilities by year. In 2008, there was only one house of hope in Turkey. As of March 2020, this increased to 152, which demonstrates the tendency toward community-based care in Turkey. Another form of LTC services is offered through "old life houses" within the community-based LTC model, which was first established in 2012. The purpose of offering this type of care is to support the participation of older people in society and prevent them from social exclusion. The older people living in these houses receive help from professionals in keeping up with their activities of daily living such as cooking, housework, and personal care. As of March 2020, the number of old life houses was 29, and the number of older people benefiting from these services was 122.

In sum, home-care assistance (see Table 1) showed a tremendous increase in terms of the number of beneficiaries. Although the number of beneficiaries in public residential care and rehabilitation centers (see Table 2) has increased over time, it seems that these institutions are not the first choice of people with disabilities. Interestingly, like home-based care, the number of houses of hope has increased over time, which may indicate that people with disabilities also prefer community-based LTC services. Also, the number of people with disabilities receiving LTC from private care centers has gone up dramatically, which may also be an indication of high-quality services by private providers.

Table 5. Distribution of care and rehabilitation centers and houses of hope for people with disabilities

Year	Residential care	
	Care and rehabilitation centers	Houses of hope
2020 (March)	104	152
2019	104	151
2018	97	146
2017	97	138
2016	93	128
2015	87	111
2014	85	84
2013	81	48
2012	80	17
2011	77	7
2010	69	3
2009	61	1
2008	56	1
2007	47	-
2006	41	-
2005	35	-
2004	32	-
2003	22	-
2002	21	-

Source: General Directorate of People with Disability and Older People Services (2020)

2.3. Benefits Package

The LTC system in Turkey is comprised of several LTC-related benefits provided by different institutions. For instance, the MoH provides health benefits, and the MFSP offers social benefits. The MoH offers health care services at home for people with disabilities and older people in need of care. Health professionals visit the sick person to follow-up with their diagnosis and treatment and to take the necessary actions in their home environment. Diseases in older people generally require LTC, which is provided by the MoH hospitals and family medicine physicians at home. Home-based health care services include rehabilitation services, physiotherapy, psychological treatment, and other medical needs (Karakuş,

2018). In 2016, the number of active/registered patients who received health services at home was 307,742, while the number of patients reached was 907,634. Furthermore, older people, people with disabilities, and people with chronic diseases are the ones who benefit from home-based health services the most. For example, Table 6 shows that 71% of individuals who benefited from home-based health services in 2016 were older people in need (Karakuş, 2018).

Table 6. Age distribution of people receiving home-based health care services, 2016

Age	% of people receiving home-based health care services	Number of people receiving home-based health care services
0-65	29	89,245
66-85	50	153,871
86+	21	64,626
Total	100	307,742

Source: Karakuş (2018).

Additionally, the MoH offers palliative care to support LTC in Turkey. For this purpose, the country established palliative care centers to offer medical, psychological, and social support to those who experience problems that arise due to life-threatening diseases, to increase the quality of life for patients and their families. As of 2016, 177 hospitals had palliative care units, with a bed capacity of 2,024 (Özmete and Hussein, 2017).

The MFLSS offers LTC in the context of social benefits to people with disabilities and older people. As previously explained, LTC services are differentiated for both groups. The MFLSS provides LTC services in residential care centers, daycare, houses of hope, and home-care allowances for people with disabilities. The number of people with disabilities benefiting from home-care allowances was 478,319 in June 2016, while the number of people with disabilities aged 60 years old or older benefiting from home-care allowances was 156,234 (Özmete and Hussein, 2017).

2.4. Financing LTC: Who Pays for LTC and Sources of Financing

In general, LTC is financed through public expenditures via taxes. However, some countries implemented a social insurance system to provide its citizens with LTC services, such as Germany, Netherlands, and South Korea. Turkey, on the other hand, finances its LTC system through its general tax revenues. Within the context of medical equipment and pharmaceuticals, LTC is financed through universal health coverage in the country.

LTC services are handled for people with disabilities and older people separately, though in similar forms. The MFLSS makes the necessary payment to the institution where care is received on behalf of people with disabilities.

The home-care allowance is estimated based on the government officer salary coefficient, which is determined every six months. For example, the value of the coefficient was 0.095247 between 1 January and 30 June 2017. Therefore, for the first half of 2017, the home-care allowance was 10,000 x 0.095247 = 952.47 Turkish Liras (TL) per month. In the meantime, if people with disabilities receive LTC from formal care institutions, whether public or private, the estimated value of the allowance would be 20,000 x 0.095247 = 1,904.94 TL (1 USD=3.5232 TL as of June 30, 2017) per month (Karakuş, 2018).While people with disabilities in good economic conditions need to make payments for the LTC services that they receive from public residential centers and older people rehabilitation centers, LTC services are free of charge for those who are not in good economic condition. This condition is determined by officials who prepare a social review report. They ask for some documents to be reported, such as payroll checks of all people who live with the applicant and a document from the Land Registry Directorate of the district of residence, showing the registration status of the people with disabilities and those who live with them.

Table 7. A summary of LTC beneficiaries, eligibility criteria, benefits, and financing in Turkey

Beneficiaries	Eligibility criteria	Benefits	Financing
People with disabilities	• Certification that the person is severely disabled (50% or more), which can be verified through the medical board report • Having difficulties in ADL without the help of others • Monthly household income per person must be less than two-thirds of the net minimum wage	• Residential rehabilitation and day care centers • Home care allowance • Houses of hope services • Home-based health services	Mixed
Older people	• Aged 60 or above • Difficulties carrying out ADL such as eating, bathing, going to the restroom, and dressing without the help and care of others • Good mental health • No contagious disease • No drug or alcohol dependence • A committee must certify social and economic deprivation • Need special attention, support, and rehabilitation due to their physical and mental condition	• Nursing homes • Care and rehabilitation centers • Old life houses • Home-care allowance • Home-based health services • YADES, providing daycare and home-based LTC	Mixed

Notes: The decision about the LTC scheme (home-based, nursing home, other) belongs to the LTC recipient. However, officials need to check eligibility criteria for the recipient and the capacity of the care facility where care will be provided.

Similarly, older people in good economic condition need to make payments toward the LTC services that they receive from nursing homes and rehabilitation centers. However, even the highest payment requested does not cover the total cost of services given by these institutions. For example, in 2015, the payment required from older people payment only met 36% of the total cost per month. Also, for older people in inadequate economic conditions, which is determined based on a social review report, services are free of charge.

Prices for private nursing homes are determined by governorships of each province, determining base and ceiling fees for private institutions to charge to their customers. Prices include food, drug monitoring, injection, dressing a wound, blood pressure measurement, simple medical interventions, diapers, and cleaning costs.

All these pieces of information indicate that Turkey has a sophisticated LTC delivery system that is mostly publicly funded via general tax revenues. This type of LTC arrangement could create problems in terms of the long-term sustainability of public finances if the dynamics of demand and supply change significantly. Furthermore, there is no LTC insurance in Turkey, either, which could potentially increase the burden on the general budget.

In the next section, we offer insights regarding the future of LTC demand and supply in Turkey.

3. The Future of Long-Term Care Demand and Supply in Turkey

In the literature, the main drivers of aggregate LTC demand are socio-demographic factors. One prominent factor is the structure of the population. Aging of the society increases the very old-age dependency ratio—the share of people aged 80 and over per 100 people of working age—which, in turn, increases the demand for LTC. In addition to aging characteristics of the society, Worrall and Chaussalet (2015) count other factors that influence aggregate demand for LTC as cultural attitudes toward the older people's care (Kim and Kim, 2004; Kim and Maeda, 2001), improvements in health and disease prevalence such as dementia (Karlsson et al., 2006; Macdonald and Cooper, 2007; Comas-Herrera et al., 2007; Comas-Herrera et al., 2011), and living status (Martikainen et al., 2009).[4]

Since LTC service provision is labor intensive, the aggregate supply of LTC is also dependent on socio-demographic characteristics. LTC can be

[4] The factors that affect the individual demand for LTC, on the other hand, include marital status (Wong et al., 2010; Woo et al., 2000), disability level (Imai and Fushimi, 2011; de Meijer et al., 2009), and time to death (Weaver et al., 2009; de Meijer et al., 2011) (Worrall and Chaussalet, 2015).

supplied by formal or informal carers. Informal carers are (mostly female) family members, whereas formal carers are paid and professionally trained workers. The supply of informal carers has shrunk during the last couple of decades owing to higher female labor market participation rates, the rising distance between parents and their children, and changing family structures (Costa-Font et al., 2015). Therefore, the share of formal carers in LTC service provision is likely to increase considerably (Siciliani, 2013).

To have an idea about what the future of LTC in Turkey will look like, the demographic projections by the Turkish Statistical Institute (TurkStat) could be of assistance. Based on the results of the 2017 Address-Based Population Registration System (ADNKS), TurkStat produced new population projections according to three different scenarios that include different fertility and migration assumptions. In this study, we present the main scenario results based on the assumption that the current trends in demographic indicators will continue.

Table 8 presents the projected median age by sex and year in Turkey between 2018 and 2080. While the median age is 32.6 in 2020 in Turkey, it is expected to rise to 35.6 in 2030, 38.5 in 2040, 42.3 in 2060, 43.8 in 2070, and 45 in 2080.

Table 9 provides information about population projections by age group and sex in Turkey for 2018, 2040, 2060, and 2080. Compared to 2018 figures, the share of people aged 80 and above—the primary recipients of LTC—will more than double in 2040, rising from 1.77% to 3.85%. In 2060, the same ratio increases to 7.08%, while it is projected as 9.40% in 2080.

A more informative piece of information regarding the future demand for LTC in Turkey is found in Table 10, which displays the projected very-old age dependency ratio in Turkey for the years 2018, 2040, 2060, and 2080. According to our calculations, compared to the 2018 figure, the very old-age dependency ratio will almost triple in 2040, rising from 2.61 to 5.98. It is then expected to rise to 11.71 in 2060 and 16.01 in 2080. This means that 100 people in the working-age (ages between 15-64) will have to take care of six very-old people in 2040, 12 in 2060, and 16 in 2080.

Table 8. Median age by sex and years in Turkey, 2018-2080

Year	Total	Male	Female
2018	32.0	31.4	32.7
2019	32.3	31.7	33.0
2020	32.6	32.0	33.3
2030	35.6	34.8	36.4
2040	38.5	37.5	39.5
2050	40.5	39.4	41.7
2060	42.3	41.1	43.5
2070	43.8	42.6	45.0
2080	45.0	43.8	46.3

Source: TurkStat (2020b) - TurkStat Population Projections.

Table 9. Population projections by age group and sex in Turkey (2018, 2040, 2060, 2080)

Age group	**2018**			**2040**		
	Total	Male	Female	Total	Male	Female
Total	81,867,223	41,059,075	40,808,147	100,331,233	50,062,203	50,269,030
0-14	19,203,791	9,855,757	9,348,034	19,333,893	9,920,395	9,413,497
15-64	55,500,076	28,044,671	27,455,404	64,623,370	32,690,027	31,933,341
65-79	5,712,705	2,612,115	3,100,591	12,507,639	5,920,798	6,586,843
80+	1,450,649	546,530	904,119	3,866,330	1,530,983	2,335,348
Age group	2060			2080		
	Total	Male	Female	Total	Male	Female
Total	107,095,998	53,151,438	53,944,560	107,100,904	53,103,777	53,997,126
0-14	18,126,086	9,301,887	8,824,199	16,813,783	8,629,491	8,184,293
15-64	64,727,126	32,825,053	31,902,070	62,873,761	31,917,923	30,955,838
65-79	16,663,366	7,970,964	8,692,402	17,347,419	8,452,944	8,894,475
80+	7,579,421	3,053,533	4,525,888	10,065,939	4,103,421	5,962,519

Source: Computed from TurkStat Population Projections.

Table 10. Very old-age dependency ratios in Turkey (2018, 2040, 2060, 2080)

	2018	**2040**	**2060**	**2080**
Very old-age dependency ratio	2.61	5.98	11.71	16.01

Source: Computed from TurkStat Population Projections.

Using the numbers in Table 9 and the current structure of LTC beneficiaries, we can roughly compute the number of very-old people to demand residential care in Turkey for different scenarios. As of 2017, the number of Turkish citizens receiving residential care either at a public (around 13,000 people) or a private institution (around 7,000 people) is about 20,000 (Anadolu Ajansı, 2017). Thus, around 1.38% of people aged 80 and above are living in nursing homes.

Table 11 provides projections regarding how many people aged 80 and above will receive residential LTC in Turkey in the coming decades. The first column of the table shows different scenarios for the ratio of people aged 80+ who receive residential care. Depending on disease prevalence among the very old, female labor force participation, or cultural attitudes, which we discuss below, the ratio in the first column could increase.

Table 11. Projections for residential care demand in Turkey, 2040-2080

The ratio of people aged 80+ who receive residential care	2040	2060	2080
1.38%	53,305	104,497	138,778
1.50%	57,995	113,691	150,989
2.00%	77,327	151,588	201,319
5.00%	193,317	378,971	503,297
10.00%	386,633	757,942	1,006,594
20.00%	773,266	1,515,884	2,013,188

Source: Author calculations based on TurkStat Population Projections.

The second, third, and fourth columns demonstrate the expected number of people who will receive residential care in Turkey in 2040, 2060, and 2080 according to different scenarios. If the current ratio prevails, the number of very old people receiving LTC at a public or private institution in Turkey will be 53,305 in 2040, 104,497 in 2060, and 138,778 in 2080. Therefore, at the very least, just because of population aging, the demand for residential LTC will more than double in 2040, will be five-fold in 2060, and will be seven-fold in 2080 in comparison to current figures. If the increase in demand for residential care is to be met by public institutions using public financial resources (as is the case now), then we might expect a significant additional burden on the public finances of Turkey.

To put those numbers into perspective, we compare the current and future very old-age dependency ratios of Turkey to those of European countries. Table 12 displays very old-age dependency ratios in European countries for 2016, 2060, and 2070. In European countries, the very old-age dependency ratio was 9.1 in 2016, whereas it was only 2.61 in Turkey in 2018, almost a four-fold difference. Furthermore, a comparison of 2060 projected figures for Turkey and European countries reveals that Turkey's very old-age dependency ratio in 2060 (11.71) is almost half of the very old-age dependency ratio in European Economic Area countries (22.7), showing that this gap will be decreasing over time.

When making forecasts regarding LTC's future in Turkey, another projection to look at is the aggregate number of people with dementia. There are currently more than 600,000 people with dementia in Turkey (Turkish Alzheimer Association, 2020). Unfortunately, there is no breakdown of this figure with respect to age. According to the World Alzheimer Report 2015, in upper-middle-income countries, including Turkey, the number of people with dementia will grow by 175.77% in 2050 compared to 2020 (see Table 13).

According to Table 14, the proportionate increase in the number of people with dementia will be 196% in G20 countries, excluding G7, a group of countries that includes Turkey, between 2015 and 2050. If we take these figures as a proxy for an increase in the number of people with dementia in Turkey, there will be approximately 1.7 million people (approximately 1.6% of the population) with dementia in Turkey by 2050. This rise in the number of people with dementia will increase the demand for LTC in Turkey in the coming years.

Table 12. Very old-age dependency ratios in European countries (2016, 2060, 2070)

Country/Area	2016	2060	2070	Country/Area	2016	2060	2070
Belgium	8.5	16.9	18.4	Hungary	6.4	21.6	22.0
Bulgaria	7.2	24.6	26.8	Malta	6.4	20.1	24.3
Czechia	6.1	22.9	23.3	Netherlands	6.8	17.5	18.7
Denmark	6.7	17.1	18.9	Austria	7.4	19.3	22.3
Germany	8.9	21.4	24.1	Poland	6.1	24.4	30.3
Estonia	8.1	20.9	24.9	Portugal	9.3	30.2	29.8
Ireland	4.9	18.7	19.0	Romania	6.4	23.3	24.4
Greece	10.3	32.7	31.0	Slovenia	7.6	23.4	23.8
Spain	9.2	26.9	22.4	Slovakia	4.5	22.3	26.2
France	9.4	19.0	18.9	Finland	8.3	18.8	21.7
Croatia	7.5	20.3	23.3	Sweden	8.1	15.7	17.5
Italy	10.5	28.4	26.8	United Kingdom	7.5	16.5	18.5
Cyprus	4.9	18.2	25.4	Norway	6.4	16.5	18.7
Latvia	7.9	25.0	27.3	European Economic Area	9.1	22.7	22.6
Lithuania	8.1	25.7	24.9	European Union	8.3	21.6	22.3
Luxembourg	5.8	16.2	19.5	European Union 27	8.4	22.5	23.0

Source: European Commission (2018).

Table 13. Numbers of people with dementia (millions) according to the 2015 World Bank income classification

World Bank income group	Number of people with dementia (millions)							
	2015	2020	2025	2030	2035	2040	2045	2050
Low income	1.19	1.42	1.68	2	2.41	2.9	3.55	4.35
Lower middle income	9.77	11.52	13.72	16.35	19.48	23.12	27.18	31.54
Upper middle income	16.32	19.36	23.33	28.39	34.28	40.43	46.9	53.39
High income	19.5	21.97	24.73	27.95	31.72	35.71	39.14	42.18
World	46.78	54.27	63.45	74.69	87.88	102.15	116.78	131.45

Source: World Alzheimer Report 2015.

Nevertheless, a comparison with other countries can provide richer insights regarding the future of LTC in Turkey. Figure 3 exhibits dementia prevalence across various countries for the years 2017 and 2037. A quick scan of the graph reveals that the prevalence of dementia in Turkey will be much less (around 15 people with dementia per 1,000 population) in comparison to the Organization for Economic Cooperation and Development (OECD) countries (around 25 people with dementia per 1,000 population).

Table 14. Estimated number of people with dementia (2015, 2030 and 2050) and proportionate increases (2015-2030 and 2015-2050) according to wealth (gross national product)

	People with dementia (millions) (% of world total)			**Proportionate increase (%)**	
Region	2015	2030	2050	2015-2030	2015-2050
G7	12.88 (28)	18.43 (25)	26.28 (20)	43	104
G20	37.47 (80)	58.99 (79)	99.14 (75)	57	165
G20 excluding G7	24.59 (53)	40.56 (54)	72.86 (55)	65	196
Rest of the world (excluding G20)	9.31 (20)	15.70 (21)	32.31 (25)	69	247
World	46.78 (100)	74.69 (100)	131.45 (100)	60	181

Source: World Alzheimer Report 2015.

These projections and calculations raise significant issues concerning the future demand of formal and informal LTC in Turkey. However, they also show that the future demand for LTC in Turkey will not be as excessive as in developed countries. Nevertheless, even if the demand for LTC is expected to be less in absolute numbers in comparison to developed economies, the rate of change in LTC demand will be much faster in Turkey. This situation poses a different type of problem: sudden excess demand. As seen from the projections in Table 11, for instance, assuming a constant proportion of people 80+ in residential care, the demand for residential LTC in Turkey will (at the very least) more than double in 2040. That sudden excess of demand brings tough challenges for the government: significant amounts of investment for capacity should be planned and/or made to match the rapid growth of LTC demand. In brief, even though the projections imply a less gloomy picture for Turkey, problems such as sudden increases in LTC demand is a challenge that the Turkish government will face in the coming years.

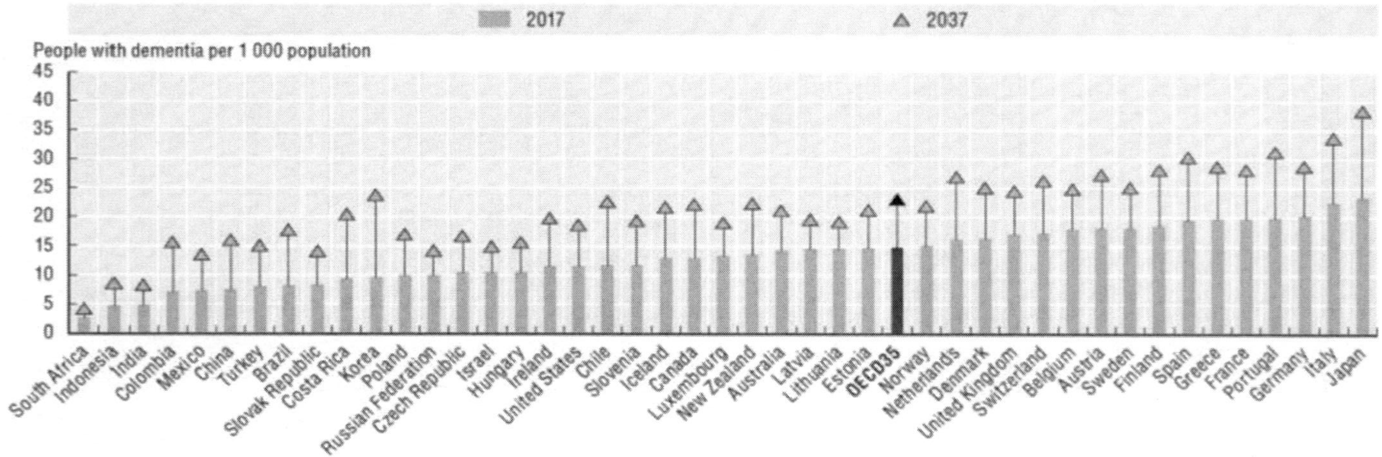

Source: OECD (2017).

Figure 3. Dementia prevalence across countries (2017, 2037).

To have a complete overview of LTC's future in Turkey, we also should look at the supply side. As in the case in many other countries, the vast majority of LTC providers in Turkey are female. According to Table 15, 85.05% of care providers are women in Turkey, whereas 66% of family carers are women in OECD countries (Colombo et al., 2011).[5,6] Therefore, the increased female labor market participation rate has the potential to reduce the size of the pool of informal LTC suppliers.

Table 15. Characteristics of LTC providers for dementia disease in Turkey (%)

Age	25-50	48.6
	50+	51.4
Sex	Female	85.05
	Male	14.95
Marital Status	Married	79.44
	Single	20.56
Educational Status	Literate	7.48
	Primary school	25.23
	Secondary school	17.76
	High school	28.97
	University	15.49
Income Status	Low	11.21
	Middle	42.99
	High	45.79
Way of Living with the Patient	Lives with the patient	24.3
	Lives with the patient and other family members	57.94
	The patient lives with other family members and relatives	17.76

Source: Özmete and Hussein (2017).

Figure 4 displays the trend for female labor force participation by age groups in Turkey. The numbers after 2018 are projected estimates by the International Labor Organization (ILO). As can be seen from the graph, the female labor force participation rate has been increasing since the beginning of the 2000s and is currently between 40%-50% for age groups

[5] Unfortunately, there is no breakdown of this figure with respect to the type of care (formal care or informal care).

[6] There could be cultural or economic reasons behind women's dominance in caregiving, which we do not discuss here.

20-24, 25-29, 30-34, 35-39, and 40-44, which compose the potential pool of informal carers in Turkey in the future (2040-2070). The labor force participation rates of these age groups are expected to increase slightly after 2030 and stagnate around 50%.

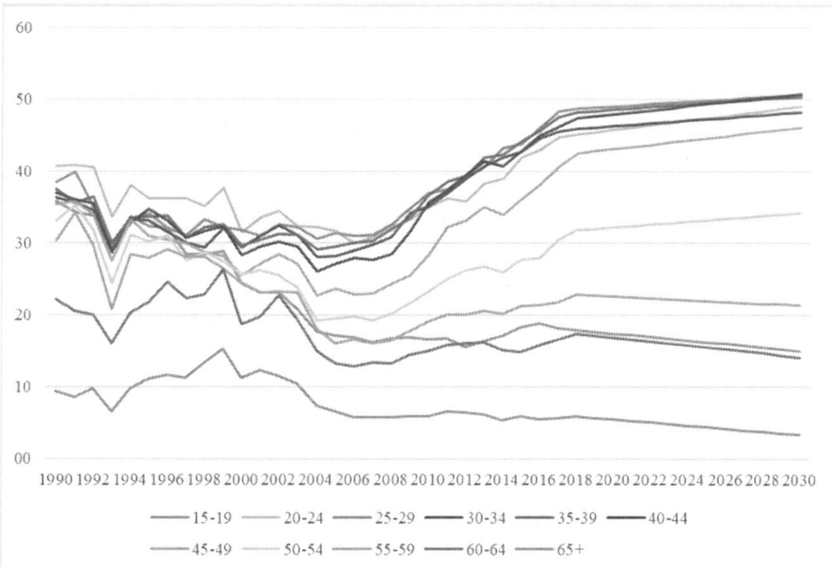

Source: ILO (https://ilostat.ilo.org/data/).

Figure 4. The trend for female labor force participation by age groups in Turkey.

According to ILO labor force estimates and projections (ILO, 2018), these shares of female labor force participation are still well below those of high-income countries, which hover around 75% (see Figure 5). Thus, the primary source of the informal care supply will not contract in Turkey as much as in high-income countries. Nevertheless, coupled with the sudden excess demand for LTC, the slightly decreasing number of informal LTC suppliers does pose a threat to the equilibrium of the "LTC delivery market" in Turkey. Furthermore, due to the population structure, the rate of decrease in LTC suppliers will be much more rapid in Turkey in comparison to developed countries, which aggravates the problem of disequilibrium in the LTC delivery market.

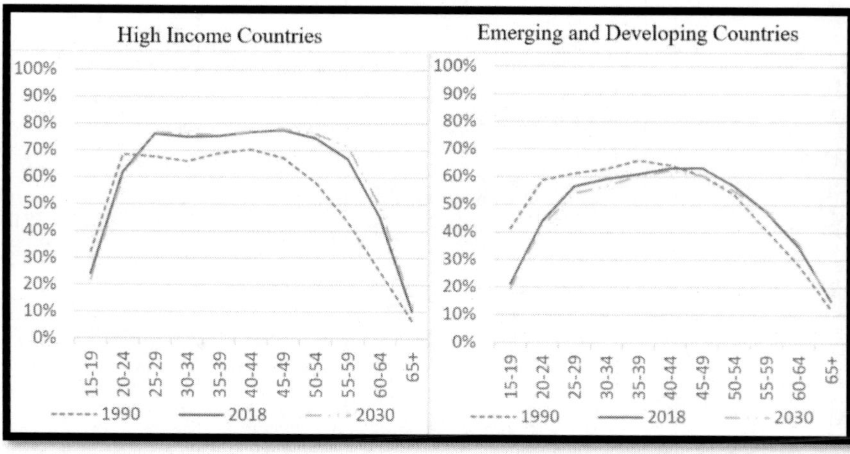

Source: ILO (2018).

Figure 5. Female labor force participation rates (%) in high-income countries and developing countries, by age group (1990, 2018, 2030).

Another factor that affects the supply of informal LTC is cultural attitudes toward older people. As discussed previously, cultural factors are among the determinants of LTC arrangement decisions (Costa-Font, 2010; Gentili et al., 2017). Cultural attitudes are especially relevant for informal care arrangements. The results from the 7th Wave of the World Values Survey (WVS) can provide some insights regarding the future of informal care supply in developing countries, including Turkey. Table 16 displays the percentage of peoples' opinions about the expression "*adult children have the duty to provide long-term care for their parents*" in selected developing countries. The ratios of people who either agreed or strongly agreed with this expression have been 79% on average in developing economies. According to the same table, the same ratio has been 38.86% on average in selected developed countries. In Turkey, 75.4% of the respondents think that it is the children's duty to provide long-term care for their parents (either "Agree" or "Strongly agree").

Table 16. Percentage of peoples' opinion about the expression "*adult children have the duty to provide long-term care for their parents*" in selected developing countries and developed countries (%)

	Developing countries															
	ARG	BRA	CHL	CHN	COL	EGY	IDN	IRN	MEX	NGA	PAK	PHL	POL	RUS	THA	TUR
Agree strongly	0	0	21.6	61.2	22	81.5	31.9	19.5	34.7	62	69.3	32.5	18.9	49.7	34.2	40.1
Agree	50.9	83.7	43.2	36.6	67.8	16.3	58.6	34.7	37.6	32.2	15.8	50.7	53.9	33.4	35.6	35.3
Neither agree nor disagree	30	8.8	20.8	0.8	3.2	1.7	2.1	24.8	12.5	2.8	8.5	10.6	11.9	11.4	17.2	17.2
Disagree	16.6	7	11.5	1.1	6.7	0.3	6.8	16	12.8	2	4.3	5.8	12	3.7	6.8	4.1
Disagree strongly	0	0	2.1	0	0.3	0.1	0.6	4.9	1.9	0.8	1.6	0.5	1.1	1.1	2.2	1.2
Don't know	1.9	0.5	0.7	0	0	0.1	0	0.1	0.5	0.1	0.6	0	1.9	0.7	1.1	1.6
No answer	0.5	0	0.2	0.3	0	0	0	0.1	0	0	0	0	0.2	0.1	0.8	0.4
Missing; Not available	0	0	0	0	0	0	0	0	0	0.1	0	0	0	0	2.1	0
	Developed countries															
	AUS	DNK	FIN	FRA	DEU	ITA	JPN	NLD	NZL	NOR	KOR	ESP	SWE	CHE	GBR	USA
Agree strongly	8.6	3.9	2.7	31.2	9	27.3	3	2.6	3.5	6.1	9.5	15.6	5.4	6	6.2	8.5
Agree	28.3	16.7	16.8	42.3	36.1	47	22.5	16.3	20.6	25.3	48.8	36.6	23.8	25.6	34.2	30.5
Neither agree nor disagree	32.9	27.9	25.4	14.1	17	17.8	44.6	30.7	32	13.5	31.9	22.1	22.1	26.6	19.8	37.2
Disagree	22.8	35.7	42	8	28.3	5.2	17.7	37.1	29.6	22.1	9.4	17.4	33.6	30.4	33.6	17.1
Disagree strongly	6.6	15.1	11.8	3.9	8	1	5	11.8	7.9	32.5	0.4	6.8	14.6	10.5	5.9	4.1
Don't know	0	0.7	1.3	0.4	1.3	1	6.8	1.2	2.9	0.4	0	1.3	0.5	0.3	0.3	0
No answer	0.8	0	0.1	0.1	0.3	0.6	0.4	0.3	0	0	0	0.1	0.1	0.6	0	2.6
Missing; Not available	0	0	0	0	0	0	0	0	3.5	0	0	0	0	0	0	0

Source: World Values Survey, Wave 7 (2017-2020), Notes: ISO 3166-1 Alpha-3 codes represent the names of the countries. They correspond to Argentina, Brazil, Chile, China, Colombia, Egypt, Indonesia, Iran, Mexico, Nigeria, Pakistan, Philippines, Poland, Russian Federation, Thailand, and Turkey for developing countries, and Australia, Denmark, Finland, France, Germany, Italy, Japan, Netherlands, New Zealand, Norway, South Korea, Spain, Sweden, Switzerland, United Kingdom, and the United States for developed countries.

Table 17 presents peoples' opinions about the expression "*adult children have the duty to provide long-term care for their parents*" in Turkey by age groups. According to this table, younger people (aged below 29) in Turkey have less of a tendency to think that it is the children's duty to provide LTC for their parents: 72.6% of young respondents either agree or strongly agree with providing care to parents, whereas 81.7% of respondents aged 50+ are in favor of looking after old parents. Thus, there does not seem to be a very striking difference between younger respondents' ideas and older peoples' opinions. Once again, these discussions imply that the shortage of informal care supply in Turkey will not be as severe as in developed countries.

Table 17. Percentage of peoples' opinion about the expression "*adult children have the duty to provide long-term care for their parents*" in Turkey by age groups (%)

	Total	≤29	30-49	50+
Agree strongly	40.1	39	38.1	44.8
Agree	35.3	33.6	35.6	36.9
Neither agree nor disagree	17.2	18.3	18.7	13.3
Disagree	4.1	4.5	4.5	3.1
Disagree strongly	1.2	1.3	1.7	0.5
Don't know	1.6	2.7	1.2	1.1
No answer	0.4	0.7	0.2	0.3

Source: World Values Survey, Wave 7 (2017-2020).

Another useful statistic to look at to have an idea about the future supply of LTC in Turkey is the number of student quotas at higher education programs dedicated to care of older people or social services. This is particularly relevant for professional LTC delivery. In Table 18, we provide information about annual numbers of graduates from higher education institutions in Turkey in 2019. The programs Social Service(s) and Elderly Care are the most relevant programs targeted at LTC. The number of annual quotas for these programs is approximately 18,000. The program Elderly Care is directly related to LTC, while Social Service(s) programs also cover other care services such as orphanage care. If we assume that 10,000 people graduate from these programs each year to work in the LTC sector, by 2040, a total of 200,000 will have been graduated. Comparing this number to the second column of Table 11, which shows the expected number of people aged 80+ who receive residential care, we can say that the additional supply of professional LTC workforce could be sufficient to meet the expected demand, which ranges between 54,000 and 773,000. Thus, higher education programs in Turkey seem to provide the required workforce for professional LTC delivery until 2040. Nevertheless, sudden excess demand for LTC for specific periods could still be a problem for Turkey.

Table 18. Annual Student Quotas at Higher Education Institutions in 2019

Department	Degree	Annual Quotas
Social Services	Associate (Vocational School)	3,738
Social Service	Bachelor (Vocational School)	438
Social Service	Bachelor (Open University)	1.795
Social Service	Bachelor (Undergraduate)	3,666
Older people Care	Associate (Vocational School)	5,505
Older people Care	Associate (Open University)	2,563
Total for Older people Care		8,068
Total for Social Service(s)		9,637
Total		17,705

Source: Authors' calculations from Higher Education Council website (www.yok.gov.tr).

Discussion and Conclusion

Although there is ample research on LTC in various subfields of economic literature, this research mostly revolves around developed countries. A significant finding of the research on developed countries is that demand for LTC has been rising and will considerably increase, and the potential supply of LTC has shrunk and will contract, which will result in excess demand for LTC. The developed countries' governments have already started taking precautionary measures to offset pressures from excess demand for LTC. However, the issue of LTC has been neglected and underexplored in developing economies. A related research question, then, is what the current situation of LTC is and what the future of LTC will be in developing countries. Do they share the same destiny with developed countries, or does a different future await them? Even though we may not fully know the answers to these questions, a comparison of the current situation and future projections to those of developed countries can give us an idea as to what we can expect.

To that end, in this study, we have focused on Turkey, which is a large developing country with a population of more than 80 million people, and we have contributed to the sparse literature on LTC services in developing economies. Having presented an overview of the institutional background of LTC provision in Turkey, we have then made a comparison with developed countries by looking at publicly available data and projections. More specifically, we have examined the projected demographic changes, have made a back-of-the-envelope calculation for dementia prevalence, have inspected the projected female labor force participation rates, and have analyzed attitudes toward providing informal LTC to elder parents.

Demographic projections point to an aging population in Turkey. By 2080, the median age will rise to 45 (from 32.6 in 2020) and the very old-age dependency ratio will increase by eight-fold to 16.01. Even though these numbers suggest that the aggregate demand for LTC will grow significantly in Turkey, the number of very old people per a hundred working population will be almost half of that of European countries, a subgroup of developed countries, by 2060.

Our back-of-the-envelope calculations on dementia prevalence show that there will be approximately 1.7 million people (approximately 1.6% of the population) with dementia in Turkey by 2050. Even if this increase in the number of people with dementia will raise the demand for LTC in Turkey, a comparison with OECD countries shows that the prevalence of dementia in Turkey will be much less (around 15 people with dementia per 1,000 population) than those of OECD countries (around 25 people with dementia per 1,000 population).

Thus, the projections of two essential determinants of LTC—very old-age dependency ratio and dementia prevalence—indicate that even if the demand for LTC will rise in the coming decades (2050-2080) in Turkey, the future demand for LTC in Turkey will not be as large as that of developed countries. However, the rate of increase in LTC demand and the rate of decrease in LTC supply will be swifter in Turkey in comparison to developed countries, even if the changes in demand and supply of LTC is expected to be less in absolute numbers. This situation poses a different type of problem: sudden excess demand for LTC. The sudden excess demand will result in acute disequilibrium in the LTC delivery market in Turkey. Resolving such disequilibria requires immediate actions that are costlier than well-planned precautions. Even if such disequilibria are addressed in advance, significant amounts of investment in capacity for LTC provision should be worked out and/or made to match the rapid growth of LTC demand.

The expected increase in LTC demand, whether sudden or gradual, raises significant issues in terms of affordability and equity. If the increased demand is to be met by formal care, are the recipients of LTC insured and protected against catastrophic (or non-catastrophic) LTC expenditures? Or, if the increased demand is to be met by informal care, will caregivers have sufficient opportunities for income-generating activities? Such questions should be addressed by policymakers in the planning of LTC arrangements in Turkey.

On the supply side, we have observed that the vast majority of caregivers in Turkey are female. Thus, increased female labor market participation rates have the potential to reduce the size of the pool of LTC suppliers. The projected estimates show that female labor force participation rates for age groups that make up the potential pool of informal carers in Turkey in the future have been increasing since the 2000s, are expected to increase after 2020 slightly, and level off around 50% by 2030. Nevertheless, these rates of female labor force participation are 50% lower than those of developed countries. Thus, the primary source of the informal care supply will not diminish in Turkey as much as high-income countries.

Another supply factor that affects informal LTC delivery is cultural attitudes toward old parents. The results from the 7th Wave of the World

Values Survey (WVS), which covers the years 2017-2020, indicate that the percentage of people who agree or strongly agree that adult children have the duty to provide LTC for their parents is 75.4% in Turkey, and the inclination to provide LTC for old parents does not change significantly with respect to age. On the other hand, the tendency to offer LTC for old parents is much lower in selected developed countries (38.86% on average). This once again suggests that the shortage of the informal care supply in Turkey will not be as severe as in high-income countries.

Regarding the provision of formal LTC, we have observed that higher education programs in Turkey seem to offer the required workforce for professional LTC delivery at institutions. However, since we cannot know exactly what portion of LTC recipients will shift to seeking formal care and whether graduates of these programs opt to work in the LTC sector, there might be sudden jumps in LTC demand that leads to disequilibrium.

In brief, the analyses in this study predict that the demand for LTC is expected to increase, and the supply of informal care is foreseen to shrink in Turkey in the coming decades, which could result in poignant disequilibrium in LTC delivery market.

Turkey currently has an intricate LTC delivery system that involves various stakeholders and processes. Currently, there is no LTC insurance in Turkey. The formal system is mostly publicly funded via general tax revenues. Excess demand for LTC in the future, as demonstrated in this chapter, could create problems by increasing the burden on the general budget, which poses a threat to the long-term sustainability of Turkey's public finances.

To take the necessary precautions to ease the expected pressures on public finances, Turkish officials must first plan for resources for LTC service delivery. To the best of our knowledge, such resource planning has not been developed by the MFLSS. Therefore, we propose setting up a resource planning system to determine the amount of resources required for LTC services in Turkey according to various scenarios. This will allow the MFLSS to have an idea about necessary inputs, such as the capacity of additional nursing homes to be built, or the number of LTC workers to be trained and employed.

One of the precautions to be taken to avoid sudden increases in LTC demand is to promote individual planning by citizens ahead of their LTC needs. This will curb the sudden excess demand for LTC and enable the government to handle the excess demand for LTC in a more effective way. To this end, the MFLSS could launch online platforms or information campaigns to advertise LTC planning processes.

Increasing the choices of individuals in their planning of LTC processes surely increases their welfare. A competitive private nursing home market is an essential ingredient to increase the options available to LTC recipients. Therefore, the MFLSS should alter the necessary regulations (e.g., about entry licensing) to increase the number of private nursing homes in the market.

Increasing the number of innovative financial products related to LTC in financial markets is another solution to increase the choices that citizens can make about their welfare. As previously discussed, there is no LTC insurance in Turkey. Likewise, innovative products such as reverse mortgages do not exist in Turkish financial markets. In cooperation with financial market authorities, the legal infrastructure for such products should be developed.

On the other hand, one quick solution to sudden excess demand for LTC could be encouraging the emigration of the foreign workforce. Currently, some foreign workers are already working illegally in Turkey to provide LTC in home care settings. Temporarily allowing foreign workers and training them could be another measure to respond to the sudden excess demand for LTC in Turkey.

To conclude, all these anticipated changes and policies proposed raise significant issues in terms of affordability and equity that should be addressed by policymakers. For instance, policymakers in Turkey should make sure that every LTC recipient in Turkey is entitled to LTC with a certain level of quality without making catastrophic payments. In this regard, one action by the Ministry to improve the quality of LTC in home settings, for example, is to offer training programs targeted at relatives of LTC recipients. The additional training not only improves the quality of care received by individuals but also increases the LTC supply if the carers of LTC recipients choose to continue working in the LTC sector once their relatives have died. Thus, they could make up for the income loss, if any, during the period when they looked after their relatives.

One major shortcoming of this study is that it cannot incorporate aging people's health status and needs into the projections, and it cannot evaluate how dependent they are. Future studies and the proposed resource planning system can overcome this drawback by studying different scenarios of aging in Turkey. Overall, more complementary studies on the design of future LTC arrangements in Turkey are required.

Finally, the lack of relevant data in LTC-related research is a critical challenge for developing countries. Authorities in Turkey should collect and publish detailed, high-quality data on LTC, which currently do not exist, to promote more research on LTC and its future in Turkey.

REFERENCES

Ağören, Veli. "Bakim sigortasi ve Türkiye için model önerisi." [Care insurance and a model proposal for Turkey] *Sosyal Güvence* 12 (2017): 1-26.

Anadolu Ajansı. *Huzurevlerinde 19 bin 818 kişi kalıyor.* [*19,818 people are living in nursing homes*] https://www.aa.com.tr/tr/turkiye/huzurevlerinde-19-bin-818-kisi-kaliyor-/727545 (2020).

Ayhan, Burcu. *Uzun süreli bakım sistemleri ve finansman yöntemleri: Türkiye açısından değerlendirmeler.* [*Long-term care systems and financing methods: assessments for Turkey*] Specialty Thesis. General Directorate of Disabled and Elderly Services. (2014).

Bal, Tolga. "OECD ülke uygulamaları doğrultusunda uzun dönemli bakım (UDB) hizmetlerinin finansmanı ve Türkiye için öneriler." [The financing of long-term care services in OECD countries and proposals for Turkey] *SGD-Sosyal Güvenlik Dergisi* 6, no. 1: 159-196.

Bolin, Kristian, Bjorn Lindgren, and Petter Lundborg. "Informal and formal care among single-living elderly in Europe." *Health Economics* 17, no. 3 (2008): 393-409.

Bonsang, Eric. "Does informal care from children to their elderly parents substitute for formal care in Europe?." *Journal of Health Economics* 28, no. 1 (2009): 143-154.

Bowblis, John R., Stephen Crystal, Orna Intrator, and Judith A. Lucas. "Response to regulatory stringency: the case of antipsychotic medication use in nursing homes." *Health Economics* 21, no. 8 (2012): 977-993.

Charles, Kerwin Kofi, and Purvi Sevak. "Can family caregiving substitute for nursing home care?." *Journal of Health Economics* 24, no. 6 (2005): 1174-1190.

Colombo, F., A. Llena-Nozal, J. Mercier, and F. Tiadens. *Help wanted? Providing and paying need for long-term care.* OECD Publishing, Paris (2011).

Comas-Herrera, Adelina, Raphael Wittenberg, Linda Pickard, and Martin Knapp. "Cognitive impairment in older people: future demand for long-term care services and the associated costs." *International Journal of Geriatric Psychiatry: A journal of the psychiatry of late life and allied sciences* 22, no. 10 (2007): 1037-1045.

Comas-Herrera, Adelina, Sara Northey, Raphael Wittenberg, Martin Knapp, Sarmishtha Bhattacharyya, and Alistair Burns. "Future costs of dementia-related long-term care: exploring future scenarios." *International Psychogeriatrics* 23, no. 1 (2011): 20.

Costa-Font, Joan, and Concepció Patxot. "The intergenerational impact of long-term care financing alternatives in Spain." *The Geneva Papers on Risk and Insurance-Issues and Practice* 29, no. 4 (2004): 599-619.

Costa-Font, Joan, Christophe Courbage, and Katherine Swartz. "Financing long-term care: ex ante, ex post or both?." *Health Economics* 24 (2015): 45-57.

Costa-Font, Joan. "Family ties and the crowding out of long-term care insurance." *Oxford Review of Economic Policy* 26, no. 4 (2010): 691-712.

Courbage, Christophe, and Louis Eeckhoudt. "On insuring and caring for parents' long-term care needs." *Journal of Health Economics* 31, no. 6 (2012): 842-850.

de Meijer, Claudine AM, Marc A. Koopmanschap, Xander HE Koolman, and Eddy KA van Doorslaer. "The role of disability in explaining long-term care utilization." *Medical Care* (2009): 1156-1163.

De Meijer, Claudine, Marc Koopmanschap, Teresa Bago d'Uva, and Eddy Van Doorslaer. "Determinants of long-term care spending: age, time to death or disability?." *Journal of Health Economics* 30, no. 2 (2011): 425-438.

European Commission. *The 2018 Ageing Report: Underlying Assumptions & Projections*. (2018).

Forder, Julien, and Stephen Allan. "The impact of competition on quality and prices in the English care homes market." *Journal of Health Economics* 34 (2014): 73-83.

Fukui, Tadashi, and Yasushi Iwamoto. "Policy options for financing future health and long-term care costs in Japan." In *Fiscal policy and management in East Asia*, pp. 415-442. University of Chicago Press, 2007.

Gaughan, James, Hugh Gravelle, and Luigi Siciliani. "Delayed discharges and hospital type: evidence from the English NHS." *Fiscal Studies* 38, no. 3 (2017): 495-519.

Gentili, Elena, Giuliano Masiero, and Fabrizio Mazzonna. "The role of culture in long-term care arrangement decisions." *Journal of Economic Behavior & Organization* 143 (2017): 186-200.

General Directorate of Disabled and Elderly Services. *Engelli ve yaşlı istatistik bülteni, 2020 Nisan.* [*Statistics bulletin for and the elderly, 2020 April*] https://www.ailevecalisma.gov.tr/eyhgm/yayin-kaynak/ (2020).

Hirschfeld, Miriam J., and Miriam Hirschfeld. *Long-term care in developing countries: ten case-studies.* World Health Organization, (2003).

ILO. ILO Labour Force Estimates and Projections (LFEP) *2018 Key Trends.* https://www.ilo.org/ilostat-files/Documents/LFEPbrief.pdf (2018).

Imai, Hidenori, and Kiyohide Fushimi. "Factors associated with the use of institutional long-term care in Japan." *Geriatrics & Gerontology International* 12, no. 1 (2012): 72-79.

Karakuş, Bülent. "Türkiye'de yaşlılara yönelik hizmetler, kurumsal yaşlı bakımı ve kurumsal yaşlı bakımında illerin durumu." [Services for the elderly and institutional elderly care in Turkey] *Ankara: Ministry of Family and Social Policies, General Directorate of Disabled and Elderly Services*. (2018).

Karlsson, Martin, Les Mayhew, Robert Plumb, and Ben Rickayzen. "Future costs for long-term care: cost projections for long-term care for older people in the United Kingdom." *Health Policy* 75, no. 2 (2006): 187-213.

Kim, Eun-Young, and Chang-yup Kim. "Who wants to enter a long-term care facility in a rapidly aging non-western society? Attitudes of older Koreans toward long-term care facilities." *Journal of the American Geriatrics Society* 52, no. 12 (2004): 2114-2119.

Kim, Hyuncheol Bryant, and Wilfredo Lim. "Long-term care insurance, informal care, and medical expenditures." *Journal of Public Economics* 125 (2015): 128-142.

Kim, Hyunjee, and Edward C. Norton. "How home health agencies' ownership affects practice patterns." *Fiscal Studies* 38, no. 3 (2017): 469-493.

Kim, Ik Ki, and Daisaku Maeda. "A comparative study on sociodemographic changes and long-term health care needs of the elderly in Japan and South Korea." *Journal of Cross-Cultural Gerontology* 16, no. 3 (2001): 237-255.

Lipszyc, Barbara, Etienne Sail, and Ana Xavier. *Long-term care: need, use and expenditure in the EU-27.* No. 469. Directorate General Economic and Financial Affairs (DG ECFIN), European Commission, (2012).

MacDonald, Alastair, and Brian Cooper. "Long-term care and dementia services: an impending crisis." *Age and Ageing* 36, no. 1 (2007): 16-22.

Martikainen, Pekka, Heta Moustgaard, Michael Murphy, Elina K. Einiö, Seppo Koskinen, Tuija Martelin, and Anja Noro. "Gender, living arrangements, and social circumstances as determinants of entry into and exit from long-term institutional care at older ages: a 6-year follow-up study of older Finns." *The Gerontologist* 49, no. 1 (2009): 34-45.

OECD. Dementia prevalence, in *Health at a Glance 2017: OECD Indicators*. OECD Publishing, Paris (2017).

Ozbugday, Fatih Cemil, Abdullah Tirgil, and Elif Gul Kose. "Efficiency changes in long-term care in OECD countries: A non-parametric Malmquist Index approach." *Socio-Economic Planning Sciences* 70 (2020): 100733.

Özmete, E., and S. Hussein. "Türkiye'de yaşlı bakım hizmetleri raporu: Avrupa'dan en iyi uygulama örnekleri ve Türkiye için bir model tasarımı." [The elderly care services in Turkey report: best practices from Europe and a model design for Turkey] *Ministry of Family and Social Policies* (2017).

Pezzin, Liliana E., Peter Kemper, and James Reschovsky. "Does publicly provided home care substitute for family care? Experimental evidence with endogenous living arrangements." *Journal of Human Resources* (1996): 650-676.

Seyyar, Ali. "Engelli ve Yaşlı Hizmetlerinde Sosyal Bakım," [Social care in elderly and disabled services] 3. *Edition, Rağbet Yayınları, İstanbul* (2013).

Siciliani, Luigi. "The economics of long-term care." *The BE Journal of Economic Analysis & Policy* 14, no. 2 (2013): 343-375.

Swartz, Katherine. "Searching for a balance of responsibilities: OECD countries' changing elderly assistance policies." *Annual Review of Public Health* 34 (2013): 397-412.

Turkish Alzheimer Association. *Türkiye'de 600.000 aile Alzheimer hastalığı ile mücadele ediyor*. [*600,000 families struggling with Alzheimer's disease in Turkey*] http://www.alzheimerdernegi.org.tr/haber/turkiyede-600-000-aile-alzheimer-hastaligi-ile-mucadele-ediyor/ (2020).

TurkStat. *Adrese Dayalı Nüfus Kayıt Sistemi Sonuçları, 2019.* [*The results for address-based population registry system, 2019*] http://tuik.gov.tr/PreHaberBultenleri.do?id=33705 (2020a).

TurkStat. Nüfus Projeksiyonları, 2018-2080. [*Population Projections, 2018-2080*] http://www.tuik.gov.tr/PreHaberBultenleri.do?id=30567 (2020b).

Ürker, Şule. *Türk Sosyal Güvenlik Hukukunda Özürlülük.* [*Disability in the Turkish Social Security Law*] Specialty Thesis. Directorate of Disabled Administration. (2009).

Villalobos Dintrans, Pablo. "Designing Long-Term Care Systems: Elements to Consider." *Journal of Aging & Social Policy* 32, no. 1 (2020): 83-99.

Villalobos Dintrans, Pablo. "Informal caregivers in Chile: the equity dimension of an invisible burden." *Health Policy and Planning* 34, no. 10 (2019a): 792-799.

Villalobos Dintrans, Pablo. "Is aging a problem?: Dependency, long-term care, and public policies in Chile." *Revista Panamericana de Salud Pública* 42 (2019b): e168.

Villalobos Dintrans, Pablo. "Long-term care systems as social security: the case of Chile." *Health Policy and Planning* 33, no. 9 (2018): 1018-1025.

Weaver, France, Sally C. Stearns, Edward C. Norton, and William Spector. "Proximity to death and participation in the long-term care market." *Health Economics* 18, no. 8 (2009): 867-883.

Wong, Albert, Rianne Elderkamp-de Groot, Johan Polder, and Job Van Exel. "Predictors of long-term care utilization by Dutch hospital patients aged 65+." *BMC Health Services Research* 10, no. 1 (2010): 110.

Woo, Jean, Suzanne C. Ho, Ashley L. Yu, and Joseph Lau. "An estimate of long-term care needs and identification of risk factors for institutionalization among Hong Kong Chinese aged 70 years and over." *Journal of Gerontology: Medical Sciences* 55, no. 2 (2000): 64-9.

Worrall, Philip, and Thierry J. Chaussalet. "A structured review of long-term care demand modelling." *Health Care Management Science* 18, no. 2 (2015): 173-194.

Wouterse, Bram, and Bert Smid. "How to finance the rising costs of long-term care: Four alternatives for the Netherlands." *Fiscal Studies* 38, no. 3 (2017): 369-391.

Yang, Zhou, Edward C. Norton, and Sally C. Stearns. "Longevity and health care expenditures: the real reasons older people spend more." *The Journals of Gerontology Series B: Psychological Sciences and Social Sciences* 58, no. 1 (2003): S2-S10.

In: The Future of Long-Term Care
Editor: Pablo Villalobos Dintrans
ISBN: 978-1-53619-263-6

Chapter 3

THE FUTURE OF LONG-TERM CARE IN THE UNITED STATES

Katherine Swartz[1,*] and Judy Feder[2]
[1]Department of Health Policy and Management,
Harvard T.H. Chan School of Public Health, Harvard University,
Boston, Massachusetts, US
[2]McCourt School of Public Policy, Georgetown University,
Washington, DC, US

ABSTRACT

Americans are largely on their own to finance long-term care, with public support limited to a last-resort social assistance program contingent on impoverishment. The high numbers of COVID-19-related cases and deaths among nursing home residents and staff have drawn attention to the poor conditions in many nursing homes, low wages for caregivers, and general underfunding of long-term care. This chapter describes this current "system" and explores how it might be improved in the future. We begin by describing who needs long-term care, how such care is financed, the different types of care providers, and the shortcomings of current arrangements, including responses to COVID-19. We then discuss immediate policy responses to mitigate problems exposed by the pandemic and conclude with a longer-term perspective on

* Corresponding Author's E-mail: kswartz@hsph.harvard.edu.

how long-term care might be much better financed and organized, particularly if redesigned as social insurance.

1. Introduction

Long-term care (LTC) in the United States (US) has long received too little attention, from both policymakers and the public. This changed abruptly in the spring and summer of 2020. At least 40% of COVID-19 deaths through November 2020 were of nursing home and residential care facilities' residents and staff: this amounts to more than 100,000 people, a likely undercount because not all states are tracking such deaths (Chidambaram, Garfield, and Neuman 2020).

The shockingly high numbers of deaths exposed the long-standing absence of enforcement of quality standards and weaknesses in the financing of LTC. Media attention revealed especially the limited resources available in nursing homes with predominantly low-income residents and the bleak conditions inside many of them. The COVID-19 experience is not just an exposure of policy failure; it is an opportunity to galvanize action to change the US LTC "system." Though people of all ages need LTC, demand will grow as the number of those most likely to need it—people 65 years of age and older—doubles between now and 2060 (Mather, Jacobsen, and Pollard 2015). Despite COVID-19, rising life expectancy rates will continue to increase the number of people who live past 80 years of age, a group for whom the need for LTC is greatest. Thus, the COVID-19 virus's tragic impact on nursing home residents and caregivers may provide the sense of urgency needed to alter the way LTC in the US is provided and financed.

This chapter explores how LTC in the US looks now and how it may look in the years immediately ahead and over the next few decades. Although the upheaval in American politics and the deep economic recession caused by the COVID-19 pandemic make any prediction difficult, the potential exists for reforms that might go so far as establishing a social insurance program for LTC, strengthening both financial and political support for quality care. To explain why reforms are necessary and how they may proceed, we set the stage with a description of the current status of LTC, first outlining the primary characteristics of people who need this care, how such care is financed, and the different types of care providers, and then highlighting how the COVID-19 pandemic has generated attention to long-standing inadequacies. We then turn to how US LTC could be improved in the future: first discussing immediate action to mitigate problems exposed by the pandemic, then offering a longer-term perspective on how LTC might be better financed and organized, particularly if redesigned as social insurance.

2. Background: Current Provision and Financing of Long-Term Care

To understand LTC in the US, it is important to focus on three key components: the people who need it, how it is paid for (primarily by Medicaid, the federal-state health insurance program for low-income people), and care providers in institutions and at home (where most people who need care reside). Just as the US does not have a single national health insurance program, it also does not have a formal program for LTC to which everyone is entitled if they have care needs. Unlike the country's combination of private and public health insurance, however, private insurance for LTC is largely absent. The public role is limited to "last resort" financing for poor people through the federal-state Medicaid program, which varies considerably from state to state. The "system" of LTC, although greatly influenced by Medicaid, is largely shaped by private decision-making and is heavily dependent on family caregivers (NAM 2016). It also requires difficult navigation among a broad array of providers to obtain paid care and administrative barriers in order to have public support to pay for it. Most Americans do not know how LTC is financed or that public coverage is contingent on impoverishment. In this section, we focus on the primary components of the US system of LTC:

who currently needs this care, how it is financed, and the formal providers of LTC services (beyond family and friends who provide care).

2.1. Who Needs Long-Term Care Services and Supports?

Just 4% of Americans (an estimated 14 million adults) needed LTC in 2018 (Hado and Komisar 2019; CRS 2019). LTC services are increasingly referred to as "long-term services and supports" in recognition that people should be supported to live as independently as possible, but we will use the term LTC for simplicity. "Need" for LTC is generally defined as requiring the help of others with tasks of daily life because of a physical, mental, or emotional condition (Hado and Komisar 2019).[7]

The number of people who need LTC is estimated by a combination of national surveys and administrative records of numbers of people receiving services in institutional settings or from agencies certified by the public insurers to deliver services in people's homes or community settings. There are several federal surveys of representative samples of the population where the surveys include detailed questions about a person's health and ability to perform tasks of daily living. Based on answers to the questions, a population-based estimate is determined. That, combined with what is known from administrative records, provides a total estimate of the number of people with LTC needs. There is no equivalent of a formal local government agency or committee that determines which individuals have needs that qualify them as needing LTC services.

In the US, the vast majority of people who need LTC do not live in institutional settings (primarily nursing homes, and facilities for people with intellectual disabilities): only 1.4 million people with LTC needs live in institutional settings. Their LTC needs are substantial enough that they

---

[7] Tasks of daily life include personal care needs (e.g., bathing, dressing), as used in the population estimate above. But in some instances the population with LTC needs also includes peole with difficulties handling routine tasks (e.g., everyday household chores, grocery shopping). Although the concept of functional impairments is common in assessing the need for LTC, criteria for private insurance or Medicaid benefits are not uniform and may include different types or numbers of impairments as an eligibility "trigger" (Wiener et al. 1990; Cohen, Gordon, and Miller 2011; MACPAC 2016, Ch. 4).

can no longer live safely in their own homes. Almost nine out of ten of them are particularly vulnerable to COVID-19 and other infectious diseases because they are 65 years of age or older.

The other 12.6 million adults who need LTC services live in the community, and almost half of them are younger than 65 years of age. They rely predominantly on family and friends to provide services and support.[8] This can often lead to family caregivers themselves incurring significant chronic health problems (CDC 2018). Many family members who provide LTC also have full or part-time jobs; in many cases they have foregone higher-paying jobs in order to provide care[9], and they lose not only income but retirement benefits as caregiving replaces paid employment (NAM 2016). Estimates of the aggregate economic value (or opportunity costs) of informal care-giving provided in the US range from $470 to $522 billion annually (Reinhard et al. 2019; Chari et al. 2015), but these costs are not included in the annual estimates of national expenditures for LTC by the Office of the Actuary within the Centers for Medicare and Medicaid Services (CMS).

The demographic characteristics of all adults with LTC needs vary by types of services used (NCHS 2019). Women are more likely than men to receive long-term nursing home care over their lifetime (30% versus 20%, respectively) (Johnson 2019), and in 2015-2016, they accounted for more than two-thirds of nursing home long-stay residents (NCHS 2019). Increasing age is a risk factor for residing in nursing homes; 44% of long-term residents were 85 years of age and older. Alzheimer's disease and other dementias are prevalent conditions among LTC users: between 42% and 48% of nursing home and residential care facilities had such diagnoses in 2015-2016 (NCHS 2019).

---

[8] By one estimate, more than 20 million people supplied unpaid LTC to their relatives in 2016 (Osterman 2017). The NAM (2016) estimated that 17.7 million people were providing unpaid LTC to relatives 65 years of age and older.

[9] One recent analysis, using data from the Health and Retirement Survey from 1998 to 2012, estimates that the median cost to well-being to daughters for looking after their mothers over a two-year period was $180,000 (in 2011 dollars) (Coe, Skira, and Larson 2018). Well-being in this study includes the implications of providing informal care to the daughter's future employability and wages.

Although evidence indicates that families want to provide care for family members who need assistance, the substantial cost of paid care is a deterrent to its use. The median hourly cost of a home health aide in 2019 was $23, and most aides do not work for less than 4 hours per day. Thus, paying someone to provide care can cost almost $975 per week (assuming the median hourly wage in 2019 and about 6 hours of work each day of the week) (Genworth 2020). The costs of living in a nursing home for more than six months are prohibitive for most people: the median annual cost of a semi-private room in a nursing home in 2019 was $90,155 (and a private room cost $102,200) (Genworth 2020). In 2019, half of all Medicare health insurance beneficiaries (by definition, people aged 65 and over or with permanent disabilities) had incomes below $29,650 per person and savings below $73,800 per person (Koma et al. 2020). For people 85 years of age and older, the median income per person was $22,750 and savings per person was just below $19,000 in 2019. Given that so many people's incomes and savings are well below the annual costs of personal care aides or nursing homes, it is not surprising that the vast majority of people with LTC needs depend on family and friends for assistance to live in the community.

2.2. Sources of Long-Term Care Financing

The financing of LTC in the US is often described as "fragmented" (Van Houtven, Boucher and Dawson 2020). It is unquestionably complicated: most Americans know little about the options and costs of LTC. People who become disabled at young ages have neither the income nor the savings to address care needs. As people get older and closer to retirement, most expect to rely on family and friends if they should need assistance for some time at home (Henning-Smith and Shippee 2015). Many mistakenly believe that LTC is covered by Medicare, the federal health insurance program for people at least 65 years of age and some non-elderly with qualifying disabilities.[10]

With one exception, however, Medicare pays only for "post-acute care" –skilled care (nursing or rehabilitation services) associated with an acute illness. Nursing home care must be preceded by an inpatient hospital stay of at least three days.[11] The care can be provided in a skilled-nursing facility or by a home health agency in the person's home.[12] The exception to the requirement of a three-day minimum hospital stay involves home-bound Medicare beneficiaries who cannot easily access physical therapy or skilled nursing that could help prevent them from being hospitalized (which would be expensive for Medicare). The beneficiary must be under the care of a physician, and the physician must certify the need for such services.[13] Beneficiaries receiving skilled care at home may also receive personal care services, but Medicare's coverage of nursing home and home health care is designed and administered not to provide assistance with tasks of daily living over a long period of time.

Only about a third of older Americans have set aside money for LTC expenses and only about one in ten have private insurance policies designed to cover LTC expenses (AP-NORC 2019; Johnson 2016). People who own their home may view the value of it as their LTC "insurance" but of course this requires selling the house, which is counter-productive if people expect to be able to obtain services at home. Moreover, in many

---

[10] In 2020, 67.7. million people were Medicare beneficiaries. About 15% of them were younger than 65 and had a long-term disability.

[11] If a traditional Medicare beneficiary has a procedure done on an outpatient basis or surgery that typically involves only a one-night hospital stay (such as a hip replacement without complications), then Medicare pays 80% of the cost of any physical therapy or other home health services under what is known as Medicare Part B (outpatient care). Medicare beneficiaries enrolled in managed care plans (known as Medicare Advantage) face different amounts of cost-sharing for any post-operative services prescribed after surgery done in an outpatient setting or involving a short hospital stay.

[12] Medicare covers up to 100 days of such care per spell of illness, but after the 20th day of receiving care in a skilled nursing facility, the beneficiary must pay a daily copayment which in 2020 was $176 per day. Care provided in a person's home has a different schedule of patient cost-sharing.

[13] Until 2020, Medicare paid for home health services in these situations in 60-day episodes; now home health services are paid for on a prospective basis for 30-day episodes. A physician must certify each 30-day episode, and the number of hours per week of such services is generally limited to no more than 28 hours per week.

areas of the country, home prices are not much higher than the cost of a year in a nursing home. Thus, the great majority of Americans, even after age 65, are not prepared to pay for LTC. If they do need formal LTC services or have needs that require living in a nursing home, they generally exhaust their savings to pay for care before becoming eligible for Medicaid coverage.

Expenditures for LTC in fiscal year (FY) 2018 were estimated to be $379 billion (Watts, Musumeci, and Chidambaram 2020), a little more than 10% of total US health expenditures. This total does not include Medicare spending for post-acute care (estimated to be $83.8 billion) or payments for LTC to careworkers who were not employees of a Medicare or Medicaid certified home health agency. It also does not include the "opportunity costs" of family caregiving, noted above.

The primary source of financing for paid LTC is Medicaid, the joint federal and state public health insurance program for low-income people of all ages. It financed 52% of the $379 billion in LTC expenditures in FY 2018 (Watts, Musumeci, and Chidambaram 2020). Just over a quarter of LTC spending consisted of individuals' own out-of-pocket spending (16%)[14] and private insurance (11%).[15] "Other" payers covered the last 20% of all LTC spending; this category includes public payers such as the Department of Veterans Affairs, some state and local government programs, and private foundations and charitable community organizations.

[14] Although out-of-pocket expenditures account for 16% of spending for paid LTC, those expenditures are dwarfed by estimated values of care provided by family and friends in home and community-based settings, as noted above.

[15] Within the private insurance category, about 60% was for people younger than 65 years of age who were receiving post-acute care covered by their health insurance policies – technically not LTC. The other 40% were payments from private long-term care insurance (LTCI) policies. Relatively few Americans have LTCI policies. In 2014, a little more than 7 million people (11% of people 65 and older and just 5% of people 55 to 60 years of age) had such insurance (Johnson 2016). Demand for private LTCI may fall further if people choose to let their LTCI policies lapse because they are worried about their incomes or think they will die if they become infected by COVID-19. Moreover, people 50-65 years of age who have been thinking about purchasing private LTCI may put off a decision on the grounds that they are anxious about their current jobs and need to preserve any savings against the risk of a prolonged recession. Further, the lingering effects of having COVID-19 are quite likely to prevent anyone who has had a bad case of it to be considered "insurable" by companies that sell LTCI.

2.2.1. Role of Medicaid

To receive Medicaid LTC benefits, individuals must be quite poor or must become impoverished due to spending on care. Many elderly and non-elderly with a disability exhaust their savings to pay for medical and LTC expenses, which qualifies them as "medically needy" and therefore eligible for Medicaid (Musumeci and Chidambaram 2019).[16] Virtually all of their incomes also must go toward the costs of care. These pathways are how many formerly middle-class seniors with only Social Security retirement incomes have become Medicaid beneficiaries.

Spending on LTC accounts for about a third of total Medicaid expenditures despite the fact that fewer than 10% of Medicaid enrollees use some form of LTC (Colello 2018; Thach and Weiner 2018). States vary considerably in both their total Medicaid spending on LTC, and LTC spending as a share of their total Medicaid expenditures.[17] The variation is due in large part to the variations in state policies on Medicaid eligibility in general and how much they pay for covered services, including LTC.

The joint federal-state framework of Medicaid requires each state to provide LTC in nursing homes and allows states to provide LTC in a person's home, typically described as home and community-based services (HCBS). Since the late 1990s, there has been a concerted effort (further spurred by federal policy in the past decade) to shift Medicaid-financed LTC toward HCBS rather than require that beneficiaries move to nursing homes to receive services. Medicaid HCBS expenditures surpassed its institutional LTC spending for the first time in 2013 and as of 2016, HCBS

---

[16] There are two "pathways" by which people with incomes above a state's income eligibility limit can qualify for Medicaid LTC benefits, both of which require people to exhaust their resources on medical and LTC expenses. States with a "medically needy" pathway cover people whose medical and LTC expenses cause their net income to be below a state-specified medically needy income level. States with a "special income level or other" pathway do not cover people unless their LTC needs are provided in a nursing home or residential facility. People who gain Medicaid via this pathway must have incomes below about 225% of the federal poverty level. Among people covered by both Medicare and Medicaid, just over a quarter have Medicaid coverage via these two pathways (MACPAC 2020).

[17] LTC as a share of total state Medicaid spending ranged from 18% to 61% in FY 2014 (Thach and Wiener 2018).

spending accounted for 57% of all Medicaid expenditures for LTC (Watts, Musumeci, and Chidambaram 2020; Eiken et al. 2018).

States have a great deal of flexibility in designing their home health benefits, causing substantial differences across the states in terms of which additional, optional LTC services are available to people eligible for Medicaid. The vast majority of states provide care under "waivers" of federal requirements that allow them to cap the number of people receiving specific benefits.[18] As of 2019, there were 277 separate waivers to expand financial eligibility and provide HCBS to assist seniors and non-elderly people with disabilites who reside in the community.[19] Total Medicaid HCBS spending in FY 2018 totaled $92 billion; waiver-related options accounted for two-thirds of the total and state plan options accounted for almost a third, with just 6% related to the required minimum services (Watts, Musumeci, and Chidambaram 2020).

2.3. Providers of Long-Term Care

Although distinctions are often blurred, LTC providers paid to deliver services vary in three key dimensions: whether they are residential facilities or providers that deliver services to people in the community (primarily people's homes but also group settings such as senior centers),[20] whether they operate on a for-profit or non-profit basis, and whether their

---

[18] Forty-one of the states (including the District of Columbia) have a waiver that permits them to establish a waiting list for HCBS services. Almost 820,000 people are on HCBS waiting lists, including 590,000 people with intellectual disabilities (Watts, Musumeci, and Chidambaram 2020).

[19] It is difficult to estimate the unique number of enrollees who use LTC because multiple waivers are now available to states to provide optional home and community based services, and people may use services under more than one program.

[20] Assisted living facilities are often included with nursing homes when analysts or policymakers discuss residential facilities as providers of LTC. We do not include them in our discussion of nursing facilities, however, because most do not provide extensive LTC services. Most assisted living facilities do not qualify as skilled nursing facilities. Instead, they provide HCBS and charge residents for such services, and some require residents who need significant levels of care to move to a nursing home. It also is important to note that the majority of assisted living facility residents who need LTC pay for services with their own resources (including LTCI if they have it). The monthly costs of living in assisted living facilities are typically too high for people who qualify for Medicaid.

organizational structure is systematically associated with poor quality of care.

2.3.1. Residential Facilities

Virtually all of the 15,500 *nursing homes* across the country are Medicare-certified (NCHS 2019), which means they must meet minimum staffing requirements that qualify them as skilled nursing facilities (SNFs). The terms "nursing home" and "SNF" are frequently used interchangeably as a result. As noted above, states define eligibility for Medicaid LTC and set payment rates for nursing homes and other residential facilities. Along with states' capacity to regulate the bed supply, this authority has long given state governments control over the size of their nursing home industries. Nursing homes vary in size. The median size in 2018 was 100 beds but the largest (at the 90th percentile or higher) had at least 174 beds and the smallest (at or below the 10th percentile) had 50 beds or fewer (MedPAC 2020, 223).[21] *Residential care facilities* are typically small (most have fewer than 20 residents). Only about half of these facilities were certified as Medicaid providers in 2016. An estimated 811,000 people were served by such facilities in 2016 (NCHS 2019, 76: Table 8); most were residents for a few months (often because of a slow recovery from an acute medical episode such as a stroke) and many were private-pay residents. Residents receive personal care and meals, and one or two staff are available around the clock. Physical and occupational therapists come to the facilities to provide services but nursing care is not provided on-site. *Intermediate care providers* are primarily for people with intellectual disabilities who are younger than 65 years of age. Most are small-group, residential facilities (Schmitz et al. 2014).

2.3.2. Home- and Community-Based Services Providers

People who receive paid (formal) care at home or in a group community setting (typically a town's senior center) may be served by

---

[21] The Department of Veterans Affairs (VA) also has nursing homes/SNFs (as well as various other residential care options) for armed forces veterans; about 7% of all nursing homes are VA or other government-run (NCHS 2019, Fig. 4).

agencies that employ and supervise different types of caregivers and by aides who are self-employed. Agencies differ markedly in whether their emphasis is on delivering more skilled nursing, only home health aides and personal care assistants, or just basic housekeeping and companion services. Medicare-certified home health agencies provide services typically needed by people after an episode in the hospital, such as skilled nursing, physical and occupational therapy. Medicaid certification of agencies is left to the states and certification standards vary across the country.

Medicaid generally pays only for home health aides and personal care assistants. Five states' programs allow legally responsible family members to be paid LTC providers. In addition, there are an unknown but large number of personal care agencies that provide primarily aides and housekeeping and companion services. Some of these agencies are certified by Medicaid but also may provide services to people who pay privately. Further, a non-trivial number of people report they are self-employed aides; the Census' American Communities Survey (ACS) finds that 10% of aides say they are self-employed (Osterman 2019).

Consistent estimates of the numbers of people employed by the various LTC providers are difficult to obtain.[22] Estimates range from 2.4 to 4.6 million in 2018, with the number depending in part on which types of caregivers are included.[23] Osterman (2019) estimates that in 2016, another 300,000 people worked as private-pay aides who are not represented in the Bureau of Labor Statistics (BLS) data and do not report earnings to the

---

[22] Surveys based on samples of nationally representative people can underestimate the numbers of people in different occupations because people who have more than one job typically report information about just one job. For example, a registered nurse who works in a hospital but also has a second job working for a nursing home will report the hospital as the employer. Surveys based on establishments (firms) can overestimate the numbers of people in different occupations when people work for more than one firm. It is not uncommon for certified nursing assistants and personal aides (and even nurses) to work for more than one home health agency or type of provider.

[23] By one estimate based on a survey of individuals, 2.4 million people provided LTC as registered nurses, licensed practical nurses, certified nursing assistants, and home or personal care aides in 2018 (True et al. 2020). The caregivers who have the most contact with people—that is, direct-care workers—are certified nursing assistants (CNAs) and personal care aides. The Bureau of Labor Statistics, which conducts surveys of establishments, estimates that in 2019 there were 1.4 million CNAs and almost 3.2 million home health and personal care aides (BLS 2020).

Internal Revenue Service (IRS); they work in the so-called "gray market." These aides' take-home pay may be higher than what their take-home pay would be from a home health agency, because they often do not report their full income for tax purposes.[24] Based on data from direct-care workers who are represented in the BLS estimates, nine out of ten of direct-care workers in 2016 were women, and they were disproportionately people of color (32% Black) and immigrants (25%) (Osterman 2019).

Direct-care workers are poorly paid. The median annual income for home care aides was just over $24,000 in 2018 (BLS 2020). The median annual income of nursing assistants and orderlies, who typically work in nursing homes and residential care facilities, was $29,640 in 2018 (this is equivalent to 143% of the federal poverty level for a person in a family of three people[25]). By one estimate, in 2017 a third of direct-care workers providing home care and a fifth of those working in nursing homes were covered by Medicaid themselves because their incomes were so low (PHINational 2020). Many employees (including registered nurse supervisors of home care aides) of home health agencies and nursing homes work for more than one agency or employer in order to earn more money. Although full-time home health aides typically work 40 to 44 hours a week, many work closer 50 or more hours if their client-patient needs overnight assistance, and they rarely earn overtime pay for the longer work-week. The work that aides do is hard, usually physically demanding, and often for clients who resent their need for assistance. Between the low wages and difficult work, turnover rates are high in nursing homes and home health agencies.[26]

---

[24] Importantly, however, they also do not receive employer contributions to Social Security and Medicare and, therefore, work credits that they will need for entitlement to these programs in the future.

[25] The poverty level income for a family of 3 in 2018 was $20,780.

[26] Perhaps because of the high turnover rates, very few LTC caregivers have joined unions to demand higher wages (Osterman 2017).

3. Ongoing Issues with the Provision of LTC Services

3.1. Quality of Care Concerns with Providers of Long-Term Care

The federal Centers for Medicare and Medicaid Services (CMS) sets the minimum standards for measuring quality of nursing homes, but states are responsible for inspecting and monitoring quality.[27] Daily nursing staffing levels is one of the key measures of nursing home quality. Recent research with more complete data on daily nurse staffing found that 75% of nursing homes almost never met the expected levels, and staffing levels dropped on the weekends, especially for registered nurse (RN) staff (Geng, Stevenson, and Grabowski 2019). The percentage decrease in registered nurse (RN) staffing on weekends was greater among larger nursing homes and those that had higher shares of residents who were Medicaid beneficiaries. These findings add to earlier evidence that nursing homes with high proportions of minority residents were more likely to be cited for quality deficiencies, especially those related to nurse staffing (Li et al. 2015). Concerns about variations in quality of LTC provided in people's homes also have risen with the last decade's push to have more LTC delivered in HCBS settings. There are almost no standardized, meaningful quality measures for HCBS care and the factors that might affect quality (Spetz et al. 2019; Harrington et al. 2017).

Nursing homes continue to have quality deficiencies because the minimum standards are rarely vigorously enforced (Harrington 2017; Edelman 2018; GAO 2019a; GAO 2020; Cenziper, Jacobs and Mulcahy 2020). Deficiencies are categorized in terms of their scope (isolated incident, part of a pattern of behavior, and widespread behavior) and severity (no actual harm but a potential for minimal harm; no actual harm but a potential for more than minimal harm but not immediate jeopardy;

[27] For an excellent review of the nursing home survey and certification process, and history of federal nursing home requirements to be certified for participation in Medicare and Medicaid, see Musumeci and Chidambaram (2020).

actual harm that is not immediate jeopardy; and immediate jeopardy to resident health or safety) (GAO 2020). Severe harms are primarily related to abuse (physical, mental/verbal, or sexual) and federal law requires nursing homes to report any indications of abuse to local law enforcement and the state agency responsible for monitoring nursing homes. However, delays in such reports and the lack of CMS guidance about what information needs to be provided to state agencies most often mean that prosecution of the perpetrator does not occur.[28] Most deficiencies are identified as causing residents no-harm because they do not involve immediate jeopardy for most residents. A frequent reason for no-harm deficiency citations is inadequate nurse staffing, which is related to poor plans for infection prevention and control.

CMS is not required to take enforcement actions for all deficiencies; for lower scope-severity deficiencies, a nursing home is usually given several months to correct the deficiency. For deficiencies of greater scope or severity, CMS can impose civil money penalties (fines) either per day or per instance, deny payment for some services, or terminate the nursing home from Medicare and Medicaid. However, these enforcement actions are used sparingly, in part because the nursing home industry has pushed back on the standards. During the first six months of the COVID-19 pandemic, when all nursing homes were quickly surveyed about their infection prevention and control measures, almost one in four were found to have violations; most were issued small or no fines (Cenziper, Jacobs, and Mulcahy 2020). As one former state chief health inspector said, "Unless the fines and penalties have teeth and significance, [nursing homes would] just as soon pay them and move on." (Cenziper, Jacobs, and Mulcahy 2020).

CMS is required to provide special oversight of nursing homes that have a pattern of serious deficiencies over at least three years, a category known as Special Focus Facilities (SFFs). Only 88 nursing homes have been on the list of SFFs in recent years. In frustration with the lack of

---

[28] The US Government Accountability Office (GAO) has made recommendations to CMS as to how it should strengthen reporting gaps and oversight of state agencies' investigations of abuse, but GAO reports that as of November 2019, CMS has not implemented the recommendations (GAO 2019b).

consumer knowledge of some of the poorest quality nursing homes, two Senators released a report in June 2019 that named almost 400 nursing homes that were SFF candidates but were not included due to lack of funding for monitoring SFFs (Casey and Toomey 2019).[29]

A major concern about quality of LTC is whether particular ownership and organizational structures of providers are significant factors in predicting poor practices and outcomes. Research from earlier decades linked non-profit status of nursing homes to higher quality of care than that of for-profit nursing homes, in large part because the non-profits had higher staffing ratios. More recent research findings have raised concerns about the consequences of nursing homes and home health or personal care agencies being affiliated with large chains of similar providers and the development of complicated and opaque ownership structures of the chains (Stevenson and Grabowski 2008; Harrington et al. 2012; Stevenson, Bramson, and Grabowski 2013; You et al. 2016; Grabowski et al. 2016; Rau 2017; Gupta et al. 2020). The consistent finding from this research is that quality of care is lower among for-profit nursing homes, particularly those affiliated with large chains that are increasingly owned by private equity investors. Of concern given the high numbers of COVID-19 deaths in nursing homes, there is evidence of a decline in the number of "frontline" caregivers (certified nursing assistants and licensed practical nurses) in the year following a private equity buyout of a nursing home and this result is based on data from years before the COVID-19 pandemic began (Gupta et al. 2020).

COVID-19-related quality concerns were highlighted by a recent analysis of staff shortages and insufficient supplies of personal protective equipment (PPE; such as masks, gowns, gloves, and hand sanitizer) for staff in nursing homes between two four-week reporting periods (mid-May to mid-June and the third week of June to mid-July) (McGarry, Grabowski, and Barnett 2020). The study found that for-profit nursing homes reported substantially higher rates of PPE shortages but not staff shortages than

---

[29] Only about ten percent of SFFs have been terminated since the program began in 1988 (https://www.cms.gov/Medicare/Provider-Enrollment-and-Certification/CertificationandComplianc/downloads/sfflist.pdf). Importantly, the list of SFF nursing homes is public on the CMS website (CMS 2020).

non-profit or government owned facilities, and being chain-affiliated was associated with an increase in the likelihood of reporting a PPE shortage. Further, the more disadvantaged or lower quality nursing homes (that is, those with a higher share of revenue from Medicaid or lower ratings from CMS) were found to have greater staff shortages, particularly among frontline workers (echoing earlier findings by Gupta et al. (2020)). As the study pointed out, these facilities have lower profit margins due to the "underpayment of Medicaid for nursing home costs." It is therefore troubling that for-profit organizations dominate the care-giving industry (MedPAC 2020, 223; NCHS 2019, App. Table V). About 60% of nursing homes are owned by or affiliated with organizations that operate a chain of nursing homes (NCHS 2019, Figure 5). By one estimate, 18 of the 30 largest corporations that operated nursing homes in 2019 managed 12% of all nursing homes (IQVIA 2019).

3.2. Financial Incentives for LTC Providers to Care for More Profitable People

Nursing homes have clear financial incentives to prefer private-pay residents and Medicare patients over Medicaid-funded residents. As noted above, the individual states set their Medicaid nursing home payment rates and the rates vary across the country. Medicaid payments are typically lower than rates charged for private-pay or Medicare patients. Private-pay patients are favored over everyone else because nursing homes determine their own rates and the types of patients they choose to serve. Long-term residents who can pay private rates and have limited nursing needs provide strong profit margins.

In October 2019, Medicare revised the formula for determining nursing homes payments, but the new formula still involves a prospectively determined rate, continuing to create incentives for skimping and under-provision of expected services. Nursing homes' profit margins on Medicare patients have been above 10% in each of the last 20 years, with one in four homes having margins above 20% in 2017 (MedPAC

2019, 210). Medicaid payment rates vary across states, but states, seeking to control Medicaid spending, typically pay rates that fall below the costs of care. Private-pay and Medicare patients are said to "cross-subsidize" patients covered by Medicaid (MedPAC 2019, Ch. 8) – albeit inefficiently, given the variation in payer mix across homes, and the lack of oversight or accountability.

Despite laws that are intended to prevent nursing homes from avoiding Medicaid beneficiaries, people who lack the resources to pay for nursing home care on their own and become Medicaid beneficiaries often have no choice but to live in nursing homes that receive lower quality ratings because they have a higher share of revenue from Medicaid.

3.3. COVID-19's Impact on Long-Term Care Facilities and Caregivers

By the middle of December 2020, the US had a cumulative total of more than 15 million confirmed cases and 300,000 deaths attributed to COVID-19 (Johns Hopkins University Corona Resource Center, Dec. 2020). As noted, between March and November 2020 more than 100,000 nursing home residents and staff died of COVID-19, accounting for 40% of all COVID-19 deaths in the US during those eight months (Chidambaram, Garfield, and Neuman 2020).[30] In more than half the states, deaths among nursing home residents accounted for more than half the deaths.[31] By another measure of the risk of COVID-19 for nursing home residents, the median case fatality rate—the number of deaths among people who tested positive (i.e., cases)—was estimated to be 15% by mid-November (New York Times 2020). This was more than seven times the

---

[30] The percentage varies among states because of early differences in reporting of COVID-19 deaths, and differences continue because some states include COVID-19 deaths of residents of assisted living facilities when reporting deaths of nursing home residents. States also differ as to whether COVID-19-related deaths of workers in nursing homes and assisted living facilities are disclosed.

[31] For example, in Pennsylvania, a consistent 68% of all deaths were residents of nursing homes and personal care facilities, and in North Carolina the equivalent percentage, which had been 60% through June, declined to 50% by the end of November (authors' analysis of state COVID-19 data).

case fatality rate of 2% for the US as a whole between March and November.

The COVID-19 toll on healthcare workers also has been high. Estimates ranged between 742 to more than 1,700 by mid-October 2020 (Grey 2020). Not all states required nursing homes to report cases and deaths of workers (and for the initial months of the pandemic, not even of residents). In Los Angeles County, California (with more than 10 million people, the largest-population county in the US), as of 3 December 2020, there were more than 21,000 healthcare workers and first responders (ambulance, fire and police people) who had confirmed COVID-19 cases since February 2020. Of these, 113 had died, with nursing home staff and nurses accounting for the most deaths (LA County Department of Public Health, 3 December 2020).

Alarming as these numbers are, the link between LTC facilities and the high case fatality rates among such facilities' residents and workers is complicated. By June, analyses of differences in case fatality rates among facilities implied that community spread of the virus was a key factor in explaining differences among areas where there were high and low case fatality rates in facilities. As one executive of a nursing home with few cases said, "It's there but for the grace of God go I." (Crimaldi 2020). The pattern of community spread and outbreaks in nursing homes was repeated in July in Florida, Texas and Arizona, where the numbers of COVID-19 cases rose sharply by late July.

But tagging community spread as the culprit is too simple. At least four factors created a perfect storm for community spread to hit some LTC facility providers especially hard in the first two months of the pandemic. Many of these facilities relied heavily on Medicaid payments for their operating revenue and did not have sufficient personal protective equipment (especially masks and disposable gloves) for their caregiver workforce or extra cleaning supplies on hand by early March. Second, facilities with COVID-19 outbreaks were disproportionately located in urban areas. As noted, the caregiver workforce is poorly paid, and in urban areas especially, caregivers often live in densely populated neighborhoods and rely on public transportation. They were susceptible to community spread early in the pandemic when it was still unclear that people could be asymptomatic and spreading the virus. Caregivers became ill from COVID-19 and many facilities were operating with far fewer workers than required, so care-plans for dealing with contagious diseases were compromised. Finally, added to this mix were well-intentioned but, as it turned out, greatly mistaken state policies in several states directed at quickly moving non-COVID-19 patients and recovering COVID-19 patients who still tested positive out of hospitals to nursing homes. The policies were intended to make hospital beds available for an anticipated surge of COVID-19 patients in need of ICU care and ventilators.[32] Tragically, the non-COVID-19 patients were in weakened health states because of issues that caused them to be hospitalized and were then highly susceptible to COVID-19 when it was introduced into nursing facilities. It is these factors together—not simply community spread—that explain much of how COVID-19 spread to residents and workers in some LTC facilities but not in others.

Further, these factors exacerbated the care deficiencies allowed by the long-standing absence of federal and state enforcement of minimum quality standards. As noted above, nursing homes with high proportions of Medicaid or disadvantaged residents are more likely to receive poor ratings. Frequently, they do not meet minimum staffing-to-resident ratios or comply with the requirement to have an up-to-date plan for preventing an infectious disease outbreak and for evacuating residents safely in the event of a natural disaster.

Policymakers' reactions focused public attention more on Medicaid's low payment rates than on the enforcement of quality standards in the nursing home industry.[33] Many states responded to the public outcry about poor conditions in nursing facilities by using some of the federal stimulus

---

[32] States that implemented versions of such policies included New York, California, Pennsylvania, New Mexico, Michigan, Connecticut, Massachusetts, Rhode Island, and New Jersey. Some states contracted with particular nursing facilities to treat just COVID-19 patients in order to isolate recovering COVID-19 patients. By the middle of May, New York and other states altered their policies requiring that nursing homes accept recovering COVID-19 patients discharged from hospitals.

[33] See, for example, "How COVID-19 Spreads in Nursing Homes," *Squared Away Blog* of the Center for Retirement and Research at Boston College, 26 May 2020.

funds from the March 2020 CARES Act to increase Medicaid payment rates to nursing homes. At least 23 states and the District of Columbia increased their Medicaid payments to nursing homes with most states simply raising their per diem rates by a percent or a flat amount (Flinn 2020; Musumeci, Dolan, and Guth 2020; Gifford et al. 2020). A number of states, following advice by public health experts, chose to contract with nursing homes to care only for COVID-19 patients and used federal stimulus monies to pay extraordinarily high rates. However, contracts included many nursing facilities with low quality ratings in the past year (Severns and Roubein 2020).

4. Reforming the Nation's Long-Term Care Part I: Quickly Increase Federal Financing for Medicaid LTC

By October 2020, the long-simmering weaknesses with nursing homes became the focus of public attention. Family members of nursing home residents, angered by the treatment of their loved ones, spoke out, forcing state policymakers to react. But the economic crisis and periodic shutdowns exacerbated states' underfunding of nursing homes, as states lost tax revenues and faced increasing demands for unemployment as well as health care protections. As of late October 2020, experts predicted state and local revenue shortfalls of between $480 billion and $615 billion through 2022 (an average of 10-11 percent of states' pre-COVID-19 revenue projections, with the shortfall impact varying considerably depending on the state's source of tax revenues) (Leachman and McNichol 2020; CBPP 2020; Sheiner and Campbell 2020). Without further federal funds, the revenue shortfalls potentially threaten a broad array of Medicaid and other services as states are forced to balance their budgets.

Partisan disagreement about fiscal relief to the states as well as the size and scope of another relief package left Congress gridlocked prior to the November election. Despite Democrat Joe Biden's presidential victory, the prominence of Republicans in the Senate suggests that large-scale relief to the states will remain a challenge, even in the face of sharply rising COVID-19 cases and deaths in November and predictions of worse to come.[34]

The Biden administration's ability to work with Congress will be critical for immediate and longer-term actions to improve LTC. The simplest policy path to addressing immediate concerns is to boost federal resources—and accountability—for the delivery of LTC. This section focuses on how that might be done. Longer-term changes would mean replacing the current "last resort," welfare-based model of LTC financing through Medicaid with a social insurance program for everyone who needs LTC—the focus of the next section.

4.1. Increase Federal Financial Responsibility for Medicaid: Raise the FMAP

Medicaid is financed through federal grants that match state spending on covered services for eligible beneficiaries. Federal Medical Assistance Percentages (FMAPs) are employed to provide higher matching rates to states with lower per capita incomes than to states with higher per capita incomes. The basic matching rate for a state cannot be less than 50% or, in FY 2021, more than 77.76%.[35]

Congressional efforts through November 2020 to increase the federal share of the FMAP formula were well short of what would be needed to cover the estimated millions of people eligible for Medicaid due to job losses and loss of health insurance (Banthin et al. 2020; Garfield et al. 2020; Dorn 2020). The first of the four COVID-19 related federal relief acts, known as the CARES Act and signed into law in March, included a 6.2 percentage point bump in the federal share of the Medicaid match

[34] Efforts to pass such a bill prior to the elections in November failed because of opposition from conservative senators. They did not appear to have an incentive to change their minds after the elections.

[35] The 50% rate means that for every dollar a (high income) state allocates to its Medicaid program, the federal government contributes a dollar. The 77.76% rate translates to $3.50 of federal funding for each dollar the lowest-income state (Mississippi) allocates to its Medicaid program.

(Broaddus 2020). In May, the House of Representatives passed legislation (the HEROES bill) that would temporarily boost the federal match to 14%, but as of early December, the Senate had failed to consider the bill. Significantly, the HEROES bill provides an additional 10 percentage-point increase to the match rate (for at least a year) that is specifically focused on home and community-based services.[36] This would provide a much larger impact on the LTC needs of people living in the community than President-elect Biden's campaign proposal to spend $450 billion over 10 years to expand Medicaid HCBS.[37] Given the vulnerability of nursing home residents to COVID-19, there is likely to be greater demand for HCBS-provided LTC in the future.

There are two precedents for Congress to increase the federal share of Medicaid's funding in response to economic recessions (Mitchell 2020). In 2003, in a belated response to the effects of the 2001 recession, Congress passed the Jobs and Growth Tax Relief Reconciliation Act, which provided a temporary 2.95 percentage point increase to the FMAP rates for the last two quarters of FY 2003 and the first three quarters of FY 2004. More recently, when the 2008 great recession caused millions of people to lose jobs and become eligible for Medicaid, and states' tax revenues dropped, the federal government increased the federal share of state FMAPs by 10 percentage points, on average, between October 2008 and June 2011 (Aron-Dine et al. 2020).[38] By June of 2020, numerous analysts made the argument that the COVID-19-caused recession and its anticipated duration would be even more severe. They urged an even larger federal increase in

---

[36] The 10 percentage-point increase for HCBS is in addition to the 14 percentage-point increase to each state's FMAP (subject to a maximum on federal spending of 95% of a state's Medicaid costs) and was to be provided at least initially for the year between July 1, 2020 and June 30, 2021. The 10 percentage-point increase targeting HCBS could be used by states to support financially stressed HCBS providers through "retainer" payments and higher payment rates (including for self-directed care and family providers); address HCBS providers' higher COVID-19 related costs such as hazard and overtime pay, emergency supplies and equipment, training, education and recruitment; and make other HCBS improvements (Park 2020).

[37] Biden's proposal for expanding HCBS also includes a promise to eliminate waiting lists for HCBS that exist in some states. As noted in footnote 12, more than 800,000 people are estimated to be on such waiting lists.

[38] The additional federal funds were not enough, however, to prevent states from adopting cuts to Medicaid optional programs, including slowing the growth in LTC enrollment via home and community-based services (HCBS).

the FMAP and a permanent mechanism for increasing the federal match rate in response to increases in states' unemployment levels (e.g., Aron-Dine et al. 2020; Fiedler and Powell 2020; Holahan et al. 2020). One of the authors (Feder) has proposed that the federal share of the FMAP also be tied to an age-based index to address the longer-term problem posed by the expected growth in the elderly population. Such a provision would ensure federal funding to meet growing LTC care needs by allocating more federal funds to states with larger shares of their populations who are age 75 and older with incomes below 300% of the federal poverty level (Feder and Komisar 2012; Feder 2020).

4.2. Raise Caregivers' Wages and Increase Caregiver Training

To improve the quality of LTC quickly, enhanced federal funding for Medicaid LTC should be contingent on state adoption of payment mechanisms that directly support caregivers' wages along with guaranteed health insurance and paid sick leave. Raising wages and improving benefits will attract more people to the caregiver workforce, reduce staff turnover, and strengthen staffing in nursing homes. Additionally, training requirements for nurse assistants and personal care aides, accompanied by federal funding directed to community colleges that offer accredited training programs, also could relatively quickly increase the supply of well-trained caregivers, further justifying raising caregivers' wages and benefits.

Given the high COVID-19 mortality rates among residents of nursing homes and the media attention to poor conditions in many nursing homes, it is highly likely that more people with LTC needs will try harder to create a situation where they can remain in their homes. This will increase the importance of maintaining and increasing the current numbers of direct-care workers with appropriate training. A recent survey of 43 states' Medicaid directors found that a majority reported concerns about reductions in the supply of such workers (Gifford et al. 2020). Thus, raising caregiver wages and improving benefits to encourage more people to become nurse assistants and personal care aides is needed to meet the future need for them in nursing homes as well as agencies providing LTC at home.

4.3. Increase Enforcement of Quality Standards

Enhanced federal funding for Medicaid LTC also should come with requirements for more frequent state inspections of nursing homes to determine if the facilities are meeting minimum requirements for staffing and safety (as well as quality of care metrics related to the health of the residents). As noted, states are responsible for surveying nursing homes to enforce quality standards, which include operation of an infection prevention and control program. But a recent review by the Government Accountability Office (GAO) revealed that in every year from 2013 to 2019, 40% of homes had deficiencies in this standard, with half being cited in multiple consecutive years (GAO 2020). Virtually all of these deficiencies were identified as "not severe" (causing harm to patients) and virtually no enforcement actions were taken. Yet, as GAO noted, failure to implement these measures is "critical to preventing the spread of infectious diseases, including COVID-19."

As the GAO and others have been saying for years, more aggressive federal oversight of quality enforcement actions is clearly required. That will require both resources and commitment. While states receive 75% federal matching funds to conduct the inspections of nursing homes that must be done every 12 to 15 months, the Medicare certification of nursing homes is funded by discretionary appropriations by Congress (Musumeci and Chidambaram 2020). Congress has been reluctant to increase those appropriations in the face of pressure from the nursing home industry to ease up on what they view as "punitive approaches" to enforcement actions. Moreover, total fines for deficiencies have dropped 10% since 2017 (Cenziper, Jacobs, and Mulcahy 2020). As a former administrator of CMS noted, "Enforcement without consequences is not enforcement at all."

Medicare also can do more to educate consumers to avoid poor quality homes. It rewards homes that receive high quality ratings, a process that could be actively employed to advise the public to avoid low quality homes. More than a third of all nursing homes received poor quality ratings (one or two stars out of five) under the CMS quality rating system of nursing homes in 2015 (Bucutti et al. 2015). The low ratings reflect deficiencies along the metrics used to measure quality, but those deficiencies often are not remedied before the nursing home's next inspection. The Special Focus Facilities (SFF) list of the worst nursing homes provides a red flag warning to consumers, but they have to know to look for the list and too often they may not have the ability to learn about it. Relying on the public to steer clear of low-star rated nursing homes to pressure the facilities to fix the problems is not sufficient.[39]

Greater state and federal enforcement of minimum standards for staffing, safety and infection control procedures, and quality of care is needed. That requires allocating more funding to inspections and taking stronger legal steps to obtain compliance from the nursing home owners and operators. One such step would be the closure of more nursing homes that have persistent patterns of non-compliance with federal and state efforts to rectify particular deficiencies. Such homes present a danger to residents. Another step would be to forbid such homes' owners (including private equity groups) and manager-operators from ever owning or operating nursing homes in any state in the future.

4.4. Improve Medicare and Medicaid Payment Policies to Assure Appropriate Payment

Reforming payment mechanisms to emphasize care over profit and reducing incentives to favor some patients over others also should be a priority in 2021. Currently, Medicare typically overpays and Medicaid

[39] In some areas of the country, the nursing homes have only poor (one or two star) ratings, so people have little choice but to reside in one if their LTC needs are substantial enough that they cannot be provided with HCBS or if there are no home health agencies in the areas where they live.

underpays for services provided. While some nursing homes claim that Medicare profits are "necessary" to subsidize their Medicaid expenses, that approach is both inefficient and insufficient. What's needed are adequate payments by each program to promote quality services that each program covers. Medicare and Medicaid cover different services because they have different objectives. Medicare's coverage of post-acute services was intended to shorten hospital stays and reduce Medicare's overall expenditures. The statute actually prohibits coverage of "custodial care" – the label that applied to maintenance LTC when the law creating Medicare was passed in 1965. By contrast, Medicaid is expected to cover services and supports to assist individuals who can no longer care for themselves.

A comprehensive plan for appropriate payment should tie Medicare and Medicaid payments in both programs to actual spending on wages and fringe benefits necessary to meet minimum ratios of nursing staff to residents, the annual updating of explicit preparedness plans and stock-piling of supplies for emergencies (and require nursing homes to maintain a greater level of such supplies), and capital improvement payments that must be used for building maintenance and improvements to ensure the safety of residents and caregivers (such as upgrading the electrical system and creating more areas where people with infectious diseases can be isolated). Requiring capital improvements of nursing home buildings has the advantage of altering private equity/corporate investors' incentives to take money out of the homes they acquire. Such a comprehensive plan necessitates more thorough inspections of nursing homes and enforcement of rules and regulations when homes are found in violation.

5. Reforming the Nation's Long-Term Care Part II: Build a Social Insurance System

Increasing federal funding for Medicaid LTC, tying payments to quality enforcement, and payment reform are necessary remedies to be implemented now. However, even at their best, these reforms will leave the country with "last-resort" assistance with LTC costs, a system that overburdens family caregivers and impoverishes and underserves people who need LTC. What's needed is a social insurance program that spreads the risk of needing LTC across the broadest possible population.

Given the current political controversy over the size and role of the federal government, establishing this program will require a major political change. The current crisis is an opportune time for pressing political leaders to move in that direction. What follows are the principles we believe should guide a new, federally funded and organized LTC program.

5.1. Principles for a New Long-Term Care Program

As demonstrated by other OECD countries' programs for addressing LTC, a social insurance program for the U.S. should be grounded in an expectation of shared responsibility among the person, the person's immediate family, and society (Swartz 2013).

Several key components for a new LTC program follow from this foundational principle. First, shared responsibility requires that everyone in the country will financially contribute to the program. Funding for the program will be financed by both earned and unearned income; the funding will not come solely from payroll taxes or contributions related to working for wages and salaries.

Second, people's contributions to financing their care should reflect people's ability to pay. There will not be any cost-sharing required of people with incomes below some percentage of the poverty level (perhaps 150 or 200%). One way to achieve that goal is to design a program in which benefits vary with income, as in proposals for "catastrophic public long-term care insurance," in which people receive benefits after an income-related waiting period (Cohen, Feder, and Favreault 2018). Such an approach could ultimately rely on a contributory approach, as in Medicare or Social Security: payments are made during a person's working years and create a sense of ownership, and partially fund future benefits. We do not advocate requiring total "pre-funding" since that would take decades, leaving the current elderly and much of the aging "baby boom generation" unprotected.

Third, stronger federal financing for and support of Medicaid remains critical, both as a new program is built and to assure adequate protection against impoverishment, whether through broader benefits or lower cost-sharing for the lowest-income population. More broadly, to that end, current Medicaid provisions that allow beneficiaries to retain certain assets (homes and assets shared by a spouse, for example) should be expanded to create an income or asset floor—say, at median resource levels—allowing people who need substantial care to retain their "middle class" standard of living.

Finally, the new social insurance program will retain but improve the current Medicaid federal-state partnership to achieve equity and enhance adequacy across the nation. The federal government should assume full responsibility for financing Medicaid LTC and set national eligibility criteria for LTC, eliminating current disparities in Medicaid eligibility for LTC across the states. The federal government also should have responsibility for oversight and enforcement of regulations related to minimum quality of care standards, much as it does now for hospitals and Medicare certification of nursing homes. With stronger oversight, states could remain responsible for inspecting certified nursing homes and assessing eligibility for services, consistent with national standards. States also could be responsible for setting certification standards for caregivers. People will be permitted to hire their own LTC caregivers but costs will be covered only if care is delivered by certified caregivers and individuals are assessed as having care needs that qualify for coverage under the federal program. If a family member or friend is hired to provide LTC services and is certified, the program will ensure that the caregiver is credited with Social Security earnings, Medicare, paid sick leave, and any other program that requires evidence of employment.

Together, these components would change the social compact currently embedded in Medicaid for providing assistance to people with LTC needs. In particular, they will shift the US away from a welfare-based, last-resort assistance program to a universal program with federal responsibility for financing and management oversight. This is similar to the LTC programs in several other OECD countries, which also have wrestled with how to share responsibility for the common risk of needing assistance with ADLs but the seemingly random risk of extremely high costs of LTC.

5.2. Benefits of a Social Insurance Program for Long-Term Care

Social Security and Medicare, the country's very popular social insurance programs, have greatly benefited Americans of all ages. Social Security's obvious benefit is its assurance that people will have at least a minimum retirement income or income if they suffer a disability. The program also has made it possible for younger generations to devote savings in longer term investments rather than having to have cash on hand to help aging parents. Medicare also has supported the development of innovative treatments for many conditions that used to be viewed as chronic illnesses of old age, such as cardiac disease and orthopedic conditions. These new treatments have provided benefits for younger people as well. Most importantly, however, both social insurance programs have reduced people's risks related to uncertainties about the future, in particular, risks of living longer than anticipated or of future inflation that would cause a person's savings for their older years to disappear. These benefits were not immediately obvious to most people when either Social Security or Medicare were created.

The task before us is to educate the public and policy leaders that the risk of needing extensive, expensive LTC poses an equal threat to lifelong economic security and requires the same collective policy approach taken in those earlier decades. Reliance on family caregivers and requiring impoverishment as a condition for public support treats individuals, not the community, as responsible to protect against this catastrophic, unpredictable risk. Social insurance provides protection for risks related to LTC that undoubtedly will change in the future—for example, those related to changes in medical therapies, knowledge of new diseases, life expectancy, and inflation—risks that are so affected by uncertainty that the private market cannot insure them. A cure for Alzheimer's disease might lower the risk of needing LTC, while COVID-19 may enhance the likelihood of needing support. Social insurance automatically responds to both occurrences, creating a fund flow and infrastructure to provide needed supports.

A social insurance program to which everyone is entitled provides a broad base of interest in making sure the program is run well and provides quality care. The program's funding will involve contributions from everyone and the contributions will be independent of any individual's own risk of needing LTC. Because the program will be a national program, people who are alike in terms of needs for assistance and income but live in different states will no longer face different rules for access to paid-LTC services. This is particularly beneficial to people who may want to move to another state in order to live closer to their children as their needs for LTC increase.

Gathering support for a social insurance program for LTC will take work. But the tragedies of so many COVID-19 deaths of nursing home residents and careworkers are fresh in people's memories in many small towns and cities. The benefits of a social insurance program for LTC and its role within an initiative to build infrastructure that supports people and families need to be emphasized by policy makers and community leaders.

CONCLUSION

The COVID-19 pandemic has exposed weaknesses in the US "system" of LTC that have been building for decades. In particular, LTC is under-funded and under-regulated – a welfare-based, last-resort system of assistance with LTC costs, with heavy reliance on unpaid family members and underpaid workers to provide needed care. COVID-19 may have upended public tolerance for so flawed an approach to so critical a need.

The high and disproportionate numbers of COVID-19 deaths and cases among nursing home residents and careworkers horrified the public.

Community spread of the virus clearly contributed to the high death and case rates associated with nursing homes. But it also became increasingly clear that society has abdicated responsibility for humane treatment of residents and caregivers alike.

That recognition should enable a new Biden administration to marshall public support for an expansion of the federal role with Medicaid and LTC in the immediate term and, ultimately, social insurance for LTC. Achieving the latter will clearly depend on the country's ability to manage the disease—especially through vaccination—and an associated economic recovery. But it also will depend on US politics. The nation remains significantly polarized regarding the role of government in addressing social ills, not only in LTC but also economic and social inequalities that were starkly exposed by the pandemic. Addressing those ills will place enormous demands on government revenues. Nonetheless, outrage over the unnecessary COVID-19 deaths of nursing home residents and caregivers has generated a political discussion about the public underfunding of long-term care. The terrible COVID-19 pandemic provides an opportunity for creating a new approach to how LTC is financed and managed in the US.

Acknowledgments

The authors thank Pablo Villalobos Dintrans, Harriet Komisar, and an anonymous reviewer for providing thoughtful comments on earlier drafts of the chapter, and MaryBeth Musumeci, Priya Chidambaram, Toby Edelman, and Paul Osterman for helpful conversations about complex issues. They are not responsible for any errors that remain. Opinions expressed are those of the authors and may not represent the opinions of Harvard University or Georgetown University.

References

Aron-Dine, Aviva, Jessica Schubel, Judith Solomon, Matt Broaddus & Kyle Hayes. (2020). *Larger, Longer-Lasting Increases Needed in Federal Medicaid Funding Needed to Protect Coverage*. Washington, DC: Center on Budget and Policy Priorities (May 5). https://www.cbpp.org/research/health/larger-longer-lasting-increases-in-federal-medicaid-funding-needed-to-protect.

Associated Press-National Opinion Research Center at the University of Chicago (AP-NORC). (2019). *Long-Term Care Poll: Are Older Adults Financially Prepared for Long-Term Care?* https://www.longtermcarepoll.org/are-older-adults-financially-prepared-for-long-term-care/.

Banthin, Jessica, Michael Simpson, Matthew Buettgens, Linda J. Blumberg & Robin Wang. (2020). "Changes in Health Insurance Coverage Due to the COVID-19 Recession." *Washington, DC: Urban Institute Report (July).* https://www.urban.org/sites/default/files/publication/102552/changes-in-health-insurance-coverage-due-to-the-covid-19-recession_4.pdf.

Broaddus, Matt. (2020). *Families First's Medicaid Funding Boost a Useful First Step, But Far From Enough*. Washington, DC: Center on Budget and Policy Priorities (April 21). https://www.cbpp.org/blog/ families-firsts-medicaid-funding-boost-a-useful-first-step-but-far-from-enough.

Bucutti, Christina, Giselle Casillas & Tricia Neuman. (2015). "Reading the Stars: Nursing Home Quality Star Ratings, Nationally and by State." *Kaiser Family Foundation Issue Brief* (May 14). https://www.kff.org/medicare/issue-brief/reading-the-stars-nursing-home-quality-star-ratings-nationally-and-by-state/.

Bureau of Labor Statistics (BLS), US Department of Labor. (2020). *Occupational Employment Statistics, May 2019.* https://www.bls.gov/oes.current/oes311131.htm#nat.

Casey, US Senator Bob & US Senator Pat Toomey. (2019). "Families and Residents' Right to Know: Uncovering Poor Care in America's Nursing Homes." *US Senate Special Committee on Aging* (June).

https://www.aging.senate.gov/imo/media/doc/Casey%20Toomey%20SFF%20Report%20June%202019.pdf.

Center on Budget and Policy Priorities (CBPP). (2020). *State Budget Watch: States Grappling with Hit to Tax Collections.* Washington, DC: Center on Budget and Policy Priorities (November 6). https://www.cbpp.org/research/state-budget-and-tax/states-grappling-with-hit-to-tax-collections.

Center for Retirement and Research at Boston College. (2020). "How COVID-19 Spreads in Nursing Homes." *Squared Away Blog* (May 26). https://squaredawayblog.bc.edu/2020/05/?cat=13,14,15,16,17.

Centers for Disease Control and Prevention (CDC). (2018). *Caregiving for Family and Friends – A Public Health Issue.* https://www.cdc.gov/aging/caregiving/caregiver-brief.html.

Centers for Medicare and Medicaid Services (CMS). (2020). *Special Focus Facility ('SFF') Program.* https://www.cms.gov/Medicare/ Provider-Enrollment-and-Certification/CertificationandComplianc/downloads/sfflist.pdf.

Cenziper, Debbie, Joel Jacobs & Shawn Mulcahy. (2020). "As Pandemic Raged and Thousands Died, Government Regulators Cleared Most Nursing Homes of Infection-Control Violations." *Washington Post* (October 29). https://www.washingtonpost.com/ business/2020/10/29/nursing-home-deaths-fines/.

Chari, Amalavoyal V., John Engberg, Kristin N. Ray & Ateev Mehrotra. (2015). "The Opportunity Costs of Informal Elder-Care in the United States: New Estimates from the American Time Use Survey." *Health Services Research*, 50, no. 3, (June), 871-82. https://doi.org/10.1111/1475-6773.12238

Chidambaram, Priya, Rachel Garfield & Tricia Neuman. (2020). "COVID-19 Has Claimed the Lives of 100,000 Long-Term Care Residents and Staff." *Kaiser Family Foundation Policy Watch* (November 25). https://www.kff.org/policy-watch/covid-19-has-claimed-the-lives-of-100000-long-term-care-residents-and-staff/.

Cohen, Marc A., Jocelyn Gordon & Jessica Miller. (2011). "The Historical Development of Benefit Eligibility Triggers Underlying the CLASS

Plan." *The Scan Foundation CLASS Technical Assistance Brief Series* No. 2 (Spring). https://www.thescanfoundation.org/media/2019/07/TSF_CLASS_TA_No2_History_Benefit_Eligibility_FINAL.pdf.

Cohen, Marc, Judith Feder & Melissa Favreault. (2018). "A New Public-Private Partnership: Catastrophic Public and Front-End Private LTC Insurance." *Leading Age LTSS Center at UMass Boston and Urban Institute Report* (January). https://ltsscenter.org/resource-library/Public_and_Private_LTC_Insurance.pdf.

Coe, Norma B., Meghan M. Skira & Eric B. Larson. (2018). "A Comprehensive Measure of the Costs of Caring for a Parent: Differences According to Functional Status." *Journal of the American Geriatrics Society*, 66, no. 10, 2003-8, (October). https://doi.org/10.1111/jgs.15552.

Congressional Research Service (CRS). (2019). *Overview of Long-Term Services and Supports* (Updated December 30). https://crsreports.congress.gov.

Colello, Kirsten J. (2018). *Who Pays for Long-Term Services and Supports?* Congressional Research Service (August 22). https://fas.org/sgp/crs/misc/IF10343.pdf.

Crimaldi, Laura. (2020). "With Diligence and Luck, Some Nursing Homes Have Kept the Virus Out." *Boston Globe* (June 2).

Dorn, Stan. (2020). "The COVID-19 Pandemic and Resulting Economic Crash Have Caused the Greatest Health Insurance Losses in American History." *Washington, DC: Families USA Report* (July 17). https://familiesusa.org/resources/the-covid-19-pandemic-and-resulting-economic-crash-have-caused-the-greatest-health-insurance-losses-in-american-history/.

Edelman, Toby S. (2018). *Special Focus Facilities: Poor Care for Residents, Limited Enforcement Consequences for Facilities.* Washington, DC: Center for Medicare Advocacy (July 27). https://medicareadvocacy.org/special-focus-facilities-poor-care-for-residents-limited-enforcement-consequences-for-facilities/.

Eiken, Steve, Kate Sredl, Brian Burwell & Angie Amos. (2018). *Medicaid Expenditures for Long-Term Services and Supports in FY 2016.*

Baltimore, MD: Centers for Medicare and Medicaid Services (May). http://www.advancingstates.org/hcbs/article/medicaid-expenditures-long-term-services-and-supports-fy-2016.

Feder, Judy & Harriet L. Komisar. (2012). “The Importance of Federal Financing to the Nation’s Long-Term Care Safety Net.” *Long Beach, CA: SCAN Foundation Report* (February). https:// www.thescan foundation.org/sites/default/files/georgetown_importance_federal_fina ncing_ltc_2.pdf.

Feder, Judy. (2020). “COVID-19 and the Future of Long-Term Care: The Urgency of Enhanced Federal Financing.” *Journal of Aging & Social Policy*, 32, no. 4-5, 350-7 (June). https://doi.org/10.1080/ 08959420.2020.1771238.

Fiedler, Matthew & Wilson Powell III. (2020). *States Will Need More Fiscal Relief. Policymakers Should Make That Happen Automatically.* Washington, DC: Brookings Institution (April 2). https://www. brookings.edu/blog/usc-brookings-schaeffer-on-health-policy/2020/04/02/states-will-need-more-fiscal-relief-policymakers-should-make-that-happen-automatically/.

Flinn, Brendan. (2020). “States Leverage Medicaid to Provide Nursing Homes A Lifeline Through COVID-19.” *LeadingAge.org* (June 12). https://www.leadingage.org/regulation/states-leverage-medicaid-provide-nursing-homes-lifeline-through-covid-19.

Garfield, Rachel, Gary Claxton, Anthony Damico & Larry Levitt. (2020). “Eligibility for ACA Health Coverage Following Job Loss.” *Kaiser Family Foundation Issue Brief* (May 13). https://www.kff.org/ coronavirus-covid-19/issue-brief/eligibility-for-aca-health-coverage-following-job-loss/.

Geng, Fangli, David G. Stevenson & David C. Grabowski. (2019). “Daily Nursing Home Staffing Levels Highly Variable, Often Below CMS Expectations.” *Health Affairs*, 38, no. 7, 1095-100, (July). https://DOI.org/10.1377/hlthaff.2018.05322.

Genworth Financial, Inc. (Genworth). (2020). *Cost of Care Survey: 2019.* https://www.genworth.com/aging-and-you/finances/cost-of-care.html.

Gifford, Kathleen, Aimee Lashbrook, Sarah Birth, Elizabeth Hinton, Robin Rudowitz, Madeline Guth & Lina Stolyar. (2020). "State Medicaid Programs Respond to Meet COVID-19 Challenges: Results from a 50-State Medicaid Budget Survey for State Fiscal Years 2020 and 2021." *Kaiser Family Foundation Report* (October 14). https://www.kff.org/medicaid/report/state-medicaid-programs-respond-to-meet-covid-19-challenges/.

Government Accountability Office (GAO). (2019(a)). "Nursing Homes: Improved Oversight Needed to Better Protect Residents from Abuse." *GAO Report to Congress, GAO-19-433.* Washington, DC: US Government (June). https://www.gao.gov/assets/700/699721.pdf.

Government Accountability Office (GAO). (2019(b)). "Nursing Homes: Better Oversight Needed to Protect Residents from Abuse." *GAO Report to Congress, GAO-20-259T.* Washington, DC: US Government (November 14). https://www.gao.gov/assets/710/702638.pdf.

Government Accountability Office (GAO). (2020). "Infection Control Deficiencies Were Widespread and Persistent in Nursing Homes Prior to COVID-19 Pandemic." *GAO Report to Congress, GAO-20-576R.* Washington, DC: US Government (May 20). https://www.gao.gov/assets/710/707069.pdf.

Grabowski, David C., Richard A. Hirth, Orna Intrator, Yue Li, John Richardson, David G. Stevenson, Qing Zheng & Jane Banaszak-Holl. (2016). "Low-Quality Nursing Homes Were More Likely than Other Nursing Homes to be Bought or Sold by Chains in 1993-2010." *Health Affairs*, 35, no. 5, 907-14 (May). https://doi.org/10.1377/hlthaff.2015.1042.

Grey, Heather. (2020). "Hundreds of Healthcare Workers Have Died from COVID-19: This Doctor Is Honoring Them." *Healthline.com* (October 11). https://www.healthline.com/health-news/hundreds-of-healthcare-workers-have-died-from-covid-19-this-doctor-is-honoring-them.

Gupta, Atul, Sabrina T. Howell, Constantine Yannelis & Abhinav Gupta. (2020). "Does Private Equity Investment in Healthcare Benefit Patients? Evidence from Nursing Homes." *NYU Stern School of*

Business Working Paper (February, revised November). http://dx.doi.org/10.2139/ssrn.3537612.

Hado, Edem & Harriet Komisar. (2019). *Long-Term Services and Supports: Fact Sheet.* Washington, DC: AARP Public Policy Institute (August). https://www.aarp.org/content/dam/aarp/ppi/2019/08/long-term-services-and-supports.doi.10.26419-2Fppi.00079.001.pdf.

Harrington, Charlene, Brian Olney, Helen Carrillo & Taewoon Kang. (2012). "Nurse Staffing and Deficiencies in the Largest For-Profit Nursing Home Chains and Chains Owned by Private Equity Companies." *Health Services Research*, 47, no. 1, Part 1, 106-28 (February). https://DOI.org/10.1111/j.1475-6773.2011.01311.x.

Harrington, Charlene, Joshua M. Wiener, Leslie Ross & MaryBeth Musumeci. (2017). "Key Issues in Long-Term Services and Supports Quality." *Kaiser Family Foundation Issue Brief* (October). https://www.kff.org/medicaid/issue-brief/key-issues-in-long-term-services-and-supports-quality/.

Harrington, Charlene. (2017). "Long Term Services and Supports Quality, Regulations, and Enforcement." *Alexandria, VA: 41st Annual Conference of Consumer Voice for Quality Long-Term Care* (November 8). https://theconsumervoice.org/uploads/files/events/Harrington_Remarks_-_LTSS_Quality_Regulations_and_Enforcement.pdf.

Henning-Smith, Carrie E. & Tetyana P. Shippee. (2015). "Expectations About Future Use of Long-Term Services and Supports Vary by Current Living Arrangement." *Health Affairs*, 34, no. 1, 39-47 (January). https://doi.org/10.1377/hlthaff.2014.0556.

Holahan, John, Jennifer Haley, Matthew Buettgens, Caroline Elmendorf & Robin Wang. (2020). "Increasing Federal Medicaid Matching Rates to Provide Fiscal Relief to States during the COVID-19 Pandemic." *Washington, DC: Urban Institute Report* (April 23). https://www.urban.org/research/publication/increasing-federal-medicaid-matching-rates-provide-fiscal-relief-states-during-covid-19-pandemic.

IQVIA. (2019). *U.S. Elder Care Market Summary*. Durham, NC: IQVIA Institute (September). https://www.onekeydata.com/reports/u.s.-elder-care-market-summary.

Johns Hopkins University Coronavirus Resource Center. https://coronavirus.jhu.edu.

Johnson, Richard W. (2016). *Who Is Covered by Private Long-Term Care Insurance?* Washington, DC: Urban Institute. (August). https://www.urban.org/sites/default/files/publication/83146/2000881-Who-Is-Covered-by-Private-Long-Term-Care-Insurance.pdf.

Johnson, Richard W. (2019). "What Is the Lifetime Risk of Needing and Receiving Long-Term Services and Supports?" *US Department of Health and Human Services, Office of the Assistant Secretary for Planning and Evaluation Research Brief.* (April). https://aspe.hhs.gov/basic-report/what-lifetime-risk-needing-and-receiving-long-term-services-and-supports.

Koma, Wyatt, Tricia Neuman, Gretchen Jacobson & Karen Smith. (2020). "Medicare Beneficiaries' Financial Security Before the Coronavirus Pandemic." *Kaiser Family Foundation Issue Brief* (April 24). https://www.kff.org/medicare/issue-brief/medicare-beneficiaries-financial-security-before-the-coronavirus-pandemic/.

Leachman, Michael & Elizabeth McNichol. (2020). "Pandemic's Impact on State Revenues Less Than Earlier Expected But Still Severe." Washington, DC: Center on Budget and Policy Priorities (October 30). https://www.cbpp.org/research/state-budget-and-tax/pandemics-impact-on-state-revenues-less-than-earlier-expected-but.

Li, Yue, Charlene Harrington, Helena Temkin-Greener, Kai You, Xueya Cai, Xi Cen & Dana B. Mukamel. (2015). "Deficiencies in Care at Nursing Homes and Racial/Ethnic Disparities Across Homes Fell, 2006-11." *Health Affairs*, 34, no. 7, 1139-46 (July). https://DOI.org/10.1377/hlthaff.2015.0094.

Los Angeles County (California) Department of Public Health. (2020). "COVID-19 Positive Healthcare Workers and First Responders Data, Los Angeles County." (December 3). http:// publichealth.lacounty.gov

/acd/docs/COVID19HCWReport.pdf. [Accessed on December 7, 2020].

Mather, Mark, Linda A. Jacobsen & Kelvin M. Pollard. (2015). "Aging in the United States." *Population Bulletin*, 70, no. 2 (December). https://www.prb.org/wp-content/uploads/2016/01/aging-us-population-bulletin-1.pdf.

McGarry, Brian E., David C. Grabowski & Michael L. Barnett. (2020). "Severe Staffing and Personal Protective Equipment Shortages Faced by Nursing Homes During the COVID-19 Pandemic." *Health Affairs*, 39, no. 10: 1-6 (October). https://DOI.org/10.1377/hlthaff.2020.01269.

Medicaid and CHIP Payment and Access Commission (MACPAC). (2016). "Report to Congress on Medicaid and CHIP." (June). Washington, DC. https://www.macpac.gov/publication/june-2016-report-to-congress-on-medicaid-and-chip/.

Medicaid and CHIP Payment and Access Commission (MACPAC). (2020). *Dually Eligible Beneficiaries: Eligibility*. Washington, DC. https://www.macpac.gov/subtopic/dually-eligible-beneficiaries-eligibility/.

Medicare Payment Advisory Commission (MedPAC). (2019). *Report to the Congress: Medicare Payment Policy*. Washington, DC. (March). http://www.medpac.gov/docs/default-source/reports/mar19_medpac_entirereport_sec_rev.pdf?sfvrsn=0.

Medicare Payment Advisory Commission (MedPAC). (2020). *Report to the Congress: Medicare Payment Policy*. Washington, DC. (March). http://www.medpac.gov/docs/default-source/reports/mar20_entirereport_sec.pdf?sfvrsn=0.

Mitchell, Alison. (2020). "Medicaid Recession-Related FMAP Increases." *Congressional Research Service Report* R46346 (May 7). https://crsreports.congress.gov/product/pdf/R/R46346.

Musumeci, MaryBeth & Priya Chidambaram. (2019). "Medicaid Financial Eligibility for Seniors and People with Disabilities: Findings from a 50-State Survey." *Kaiser Family Foundation Issue Brief* (June). https://www.kff.org/medicaid/issue-brief/medicaid-financial-eligibility-for-seniors-and-people-with-disabilities-findings-from-a-50-state-survey/.

Musumeci, MaryBeth & Priya Chidambaram. (2020). "Key Questions About Nursing Home Regulation and Oversight in the Wake of COVID-19." *Kaiser Family Foundation Issue Brief* (August 3). https://www.kff.org/coronavirus-covid-19/issue-brief/key-questions-about-nursing-home-regulation-and-oversight-in-the-wake-of-covid-19/.

Musumeci, MaryBeth, Rachel Dolan & Madeline Guth. (2020). "State Actions to Sustain Medicaid Long-Term Services and Supports During COVID-19." *Kaiser Family Foundation Issue Brief* (August 26). https://www.kff.org/medicaid/issue-brief/state-actions-to-sustain-medicaid-long-term-services-and-supports-during-covid-19/.

National Academies of Sciences, Engineering, and Medicine (NAM). (2016). *Families Caring for an Aging America*. Washington, DC: The National Academies Press. https://doi.org/10.17226/23606.

National Center for Health Statistics (NCHS), US Department of Health and Human Services. (2019). *Long-term Care Providers and Services Users in the United States, 2015-2016*. Series 3, no. 43 (February). DHHS Pub. no. 2019-1427. https://www.cdc.gov/nchs/data/series/sr_03/sr03_43-508.pdf.

New York Times. (2020). "About 37% of U.S. Coronavirus Deaths Are Linked to Nursing Homes." *New York Times Interactive Website* (updated November 20). https://nyti.ms/31mkr1B. [Accessed on December 7, 2020].

Osterman, Paul. (2017). *Who Will Care for Us?: Long-Term Care and the Long-Term Care Workforce*. New York, NY: Russell Sage Foundation Press.

Osterman, Paul. (2019). "Improving Job Quality in Long-Term Care." In *Creating Good Jobs*, edited by Paul Osterman, Chapter 3, 115-43. Cambridge, MA: MIT Press.

Park, Edwin. (2020). *HEROES Act Includes Other Provisions Strengthening Medicaid and CHIP*. Washington, DC: Georgetown University Health Policy Institute (May 14). https:// ccf.

georgetown.edu/2020/05/14/heroes-act-includes-other-provisions-strengthening-medicaid-and-chip/.

PHINational.org. (2020). "Workforce Data Center." New York, NY. https://phinational.org/policy-research/workforce-data-center/#tab=National+Data&natvar=Public+Assistance.

Rau, Jordan. (2017). "Care Suffers as More Nursing Homes Feed Money into Corporate Webs." *New York Times* (January 2). https://www.nytimes.com/2018/01/02/business/nursing-homes-care-corporate.html.

Reinhard, Susan C., Lynn Friss Feinberg, Air Houser, Rita Choula & Molly Evans. (2019). *Valuing the Invaluable: 2019 Update.* Washington, DC: AARP Public Policy Institute. http:// www.advancingstates.org/sites/nasuad/files/valuing-the-invaluable-2019-update-charting-a-path-forward.doi_.10.26419-2Fppi.00082.001.pdf.

Schmitz, Robert, Victoria Peebles, Rosemary Borck & Dean Miller. (2014). *Medicaid-Financed Institutional Services: Patterns of Care for Residents of Nursing Homes and Intermediate Care Facilities for Individuals with Intellectual Disabilities in 2008 and 2009.* US Department of Health and Human Services, Office of the Assistant Secretary for Planning and Evaluation. (May). https://aspe.hhs.gov/system/files/pdf/137851/CarePatt.pdf.

Severns, Maggie & Rachel Roubein. (2020). "States Prod Nursing Homes to Take More Covid-19 Patients." *Politico.com* (June 4). https://www.politico.com/news/2020/06/04/states-nursing-homes-coronavirus-302134.

Sheiner, Louise & Sophia Campbell. (2020). *How Much is COVID-19 Hurting State and Local Revenues?* Washington, DC: Brookings Institution (September 24). https://www.brookings.edu/blog/up-front/2020/09/24/how-much-is-covid-19-hurting-state-and-local-revenues/.

Spetz, Joanne, Robyn I. Stone, Susan A. Chapman & Natasha Bryant. (2019). "Home and Community-Based Workforce for Patients with Serious Illness Requires Support to Meet Growing Needs." *Health Affairs*, 38, no. 6, 902-9, (June). https://DOI.org/10.1377/hlthaff.2019.00021.

Stevenson, David G. & David C. Grabowski. (2008). "Private Equity Investment and Nursing Home Care: Is It A Big Deal?" *Health Affairs*, 27, no. 5, 1399-408 (September/October). https://DOI.org/10.1377/hlthaff.27.5.1399.

Stevenson, David G., Jeffrey S. Bramson & David C. Grabowski. (2013). "Nursing Home Ownership Trends and Their Impact on Quality of Care: A Study Using Detailed Ownership Data from Texas." *Journal of Aging & Social Policy*, 25, no. 1, 30-47 (published online December 20, 2012). https://DOI.org/10.1080/08959420.2012.705702.

Swartz, Katherine. (2013). "Searching for a Balance of Responsibilities: OECD Countries' Changing Elderly Assistance Policies," *Annual Review of Public Health*, 34, 397-412. https://doi.org/10.1146/annurev-publhealth-031912-114505.

Thach, Nga T. & Joshua M. Wiener. (2018). *An Overview of Long-Term Services and Supports and Medicaid: Final Report*. US Department of Health and Human Services, Office of the Assistant Secretary for Planning and Evaluation. (May). https://aspe.hhs.gov/basic-report/overview-long-term-services-and-supports-and-medicaid-final-report.

True, Sarah, Juliette Cubanski, Rachel Garfield, Matthew Rae, Gary Claxton, Priya Chidambaram & Kendal Orgera. (2020). "COVID-19 and Workers at Risk: Examining the Long-Term Care Workforce." *Kaiser Family Foundation Issue Brief* (April 23). https://www.kff.org/coronavirus-covid-19/issue-brief/covid-19-and-workers-at-risk-examining-the-long-term-care-workforce/.

Van Houtven, Courtney H., Nathan A. Boucher & Walter D. Dawson. (2020). *Impact of the COVID-19 Outbreak on Long-Term Care in the United States*. International Long Term Care Policy Network. (April 24). https://ltccovid.org/wp-content/uploads/2020/04/USA-LTC-COVID-situation-report-24-April-2020.pdf.

Watts, Molly O'Malley, MaryBeth Musumeci & Priya Chidambaram. (2020). "Medicaid Home and Community-Based Services Enrollment and Spending." *Kaiser Family Foundation Issue Brief* (February). https://www.kff.org/medicaid/issue-brief/medicaid-home-and-community-based-services-enrollment-and-spending/.

Wiener, Joshua M., Raymond Hanley, Robert Clark & Joan F. Van Nostrand. (1990). "Measuring the Activities of Daily Living: Comparisons Across National Surveys." US Department of Health and Human Services, Office of the Assistant Secretary for Planning and Evaluation. Also published in *Journal of Gerontology: SOCIAL SCIENCES*, 45, no. 6, S229-37. https://aspe.hhs.gov/system/files/pdf/74346/meacmpes.pdf.

You, Kai, Yue Li, Orna Intrator, David Stevenson, Richard Hirth, David Grabowski & Jane Banaszak-Holl. (2016). "Do Nursing Home Chain Size and Proprietary Status Affect Experiences with Care?" *Medical Care*, 54, no. 3, 229-34 (March). https://DOI.org/10.1097/MLR.0000000000000479.

In: The Future of Long-Term Care
Editor: Pablo Villalobos Dintrans
ISBN: 978-1-53619-263-6

Chapter 4

TOWARDS A BETTER UNDERSTANDING OF THE LONG-TERM CARE NEEDS OF OLDER PEOPLE IN GHANA

Kofi Awuviry-Newton[1,*], Meredith Tavener[2], Kylie Wales[3] and Julie Byles[1]

[1]Research Centre for Generational Health and Ageing, Faculty of Health and Medicine, Hunter Medical Research Institutes, The University of Newcastle, Australia

[2]School of Medicine and Public Health, Faculty of Health and Medicine, The University of Newcastle, Australia

[3]School of Health Sciences, Faculty of Health and Medicine, The University of Newcastle, Australia

ABSTRACT

Ghana is one of the countries in sub-Saharan Africa experiencing population ageing spanning from decreasing death and delayed mortality. Even though this development is a success, it raises concerns for the long-term care (LTC) needs of older people in Ghana.

---

* Corresponding Author's E-mail: newscous@gmail.com.

The overall aim of this chapter is to discuss the LTC needs of older people as a multifactorial concept, drawing attention to the need for multiple interventions to prepare for and sustain LTC for older people in Ghana. This chapter first sets the scene for contextual understanding by discussing the evolution of familial care for older people in the country. It then draws attention to the urgent issue of LTC for older people in light of increasing care needs of older people, the burden on caregivers and the support systems that exist in the Ghanaian context, including care institutions. Finally, the chapter offers some practical recommendations for preparing for, enacting, implementing, and sustaining LTC systems and arrangements unique to older people's needs in the Ghanaian context.

1. Introduction

This chapter was motivated by the authors' experiences working in the field with caregivers and older people (people aged 60 years or older) between 2017 and 2018 in Ghana. During this period, the burden of caregiving on older people and caregivers themselves became clear in their narratives. In the authors' quest to understand the long-term care (LTC) needs of older people, it appeared that the subject of LTC is intertwined with various essential factors. These relevant factors include the care needs of older people, burden on caregivers, and systemic factors in Ghana. Understanding these factors is essential to understanding LTC overall because the failure or success in these areas will have a direct correlation with the LTC of older people in the country. To explain the LTC needs of older people in the country, we present evidence of population ageing in Ghana in the context of sub-Saharan Africa and the rest of the world.

The world's population is growing older owing to a general reduction in birth rate and increase in life expectancy (He, Goodkind, & Kowal, 2016). Despite this available projection of growth, there is variation by continent. The sub-Saharan Africa region, of which Ghana is a part, is comparatively younger than the rest of the world's seven continents (United Nations, Department of Economic and Social Affairs, & Division, 2019a). The fertility rate in this region remains high, at 4.6 live births per woman, higher than the global fertility rate of 2.5 live births per women in 2019 (United Nations, Department of Economic and Social Affairs, &

Division, 2019b). While there is a projection of a decrease in the world's fertility rate by 2050 (2.2 live births per woman) and 2100 (1.9 live births per woman), Figure 1 shows that the largest reduction in average total fertility is expected to occur in sub-Saharan Africa (United Nations et al., 2019b).

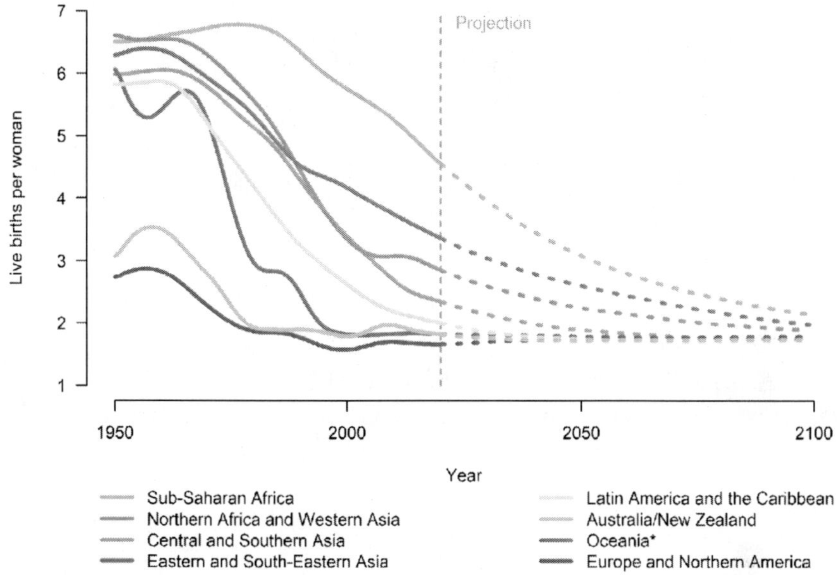

Source: United Nations (2019a).

* Excluding Australia and New Zealand.

Figure 1. Average total fertility rates by continent (1950-2100).

At the same time, there has been a marked improvement in life expectancy at birth since 1960 in sub-Saharan Africa. Life expectancy in the sub-Saharan Africa region increased from approximately 49.4 years in 1960 to 61.1 years in 2019 (United Nations et al., 2019a). Comparatively, this 11.7-year increase recorded in sub-Saharan Africa is higher than the 11-year increase recorded in Central and southern Asia during the same period (United Nations et al., 2019b). Life expectancy in sub-Saharan Africa is the lowest when compared to the rest of the continents, which is significant and worthy of noting as far as population ageing is concerned.

Comparing sub-Saharan Africa's birth rates and life expectancy with those in Ghana, it can be inferred that Ghana's challenges are more significant, requiring the country to better prepare for the challenges that come with population ageing, particularly in LTC for older people. The Ghanaian population began growing older from 1960, primarily due to the reduction in birth rates and delayed mortality (Biritwum et al., 2013a). Ghana's birth rates have steadily decreased from 6.8 live births per woman in 1960 to 3.9 in 2019, with a further projected decline to 2.8 live births per woman by 2050. This projected reduction will be higher than the anticipated decline in birth rates in high-income countries (Orji, Rao, Thompson, & Brieger, 2017; United Nations et al., 2019b). Ghana's older population increased from 273,400 (4.1% of the population) to 169 million (5.5% of the population) in the 60 years between 1960 and 2020. The pace of ageing is set to increase dramatically, with the percentage of older people projected to reach 9.8% by 2050 (United Nations, 2017).

It is a significant achievement for a developing country like Ghana to observe this improvement. This achievement implies that there are improvements in health, leading to an increasing life expectancy for Ghanaians. For example, the life expectancy at birth of 46.9 years in 1960 transformed to 63.7 years in 2020, with further increases projected to approximately 70 years by 2050 and 76.2 by 2100 (United Nations et al., 2019a). As life expectancy increases, meeting the LTC needs of older people will become a necessity for Ghana, as recommended by the World Health Organisation (2017). It appears that the LTC needs of older people are intertwined with the status of older people's functional needs, the lived experiences of caregivers, and the status of state provisions to mitigate LTC challenges that are the result of population ageing. According to the World Health Organisation (2017), LTC refers to the series of activities provided to ensure that older people that have (or potentially developing) significant, constant diminishing of their intrinsic capacities are able to maintain a level of functional ability. Satisfying these activities are necessary to ensure that older people' LTC needs are met in line with their basic rights, fundamental freedoms, and human dignity (World Health Organisation, 2017). Since fulfilling these LTC aims is complex, it requires Ghanaians to have a thorough understanding of the care needs of older people, the burden this places on caregivers, and the state's level of preparedness to meet the LTC needs of older people.

2. Understanding the Long-Term Care Needs of Older People

2.1. Understanding the Needs of Older People

LTC is generally crucial for people with disabilities who need support in accomplishing their daily life activities, in line with their basic human rights and freedoms (World Health Organisation, 2017). Among the populations who may need LTC are older people, which follows from general population ageing and its accompanying challenges relating to LTC. Though some older people in Ghana perform personal care for others (Awuviry-Newton, Ofori-Dua, & Newton, 2020b), it is imperative to understand the care needs of older people to understand their present and future LTC needs. Ghanaian older people's care needs can be better understood from a holistic perspective. They are multifactorial, spanning from personal, health, societal participation and environmental needs (Awuviry-Newton, Wales, Tavener, & Byles, 2020d). In this case, one would be mistaken to look at the care needs of older people from a health perspective only, such as for older people suffering from a chronic condition or illness affecting their day-to-day activities. Holistically, in the Ghanaian context and everywhere, factors potentially increasing older people's care needs also include environmental impediments, such as the lack of social networks or the absence of assistive devices.

In terms of health, oldest people in Ghana report experiencing some functional disability, as measured by the WHODAS (v2) score in the Biritwum et al. (2016) study. Specifically, older people experience difficulties in areas such as toileting, household chores, and participation (Amosun, Nyante, & Wiredu, 2013; Awuviry-Newton, Tavener, Wales, & Byles, 2020c; Biritwum et al., 2016; Calys-Tagoe et al., 2014; Peltzer et al., 2014). For example, Biritwum et al. (2016) report that about nine out of ten older people experience some functional disability across items assessing cognition, mobility, self-care, getting along with friends, life activities and participation in society in Ghana. Older people aged 90 years or older are more likely to report poor health (Debpuur, Welaga, Wak, & Hodgson, 2010). Similarly, people aged 60 or older experience restrictions with participation in voluntary work, including childcare. They admit having difficulties moving around inside their home and managing work (Amosun et al., 2013). The prevalence of toileting difficulties among older people in Ghana reaches 22% (Awuviry-Newton, Tavener, Wales, Kowal, & Byles, 2019). Concerning the necessary activities of daily living, older people report having trouble with climbing stairs without resting, carrying things, transferring and eating. In most of the functional disability categories, older women experience more functional difficulties than older men in Ghana (Awuviry-Newton et al., 2019; Debpuur et al., 2010).

Evidence of the experiences of older people regarding their functional disabilities is limited in Ghana; however, available evidence of older peoples' narratives enlightens our understanding of the LTC needs of older people in the country (Awuviry-Newton et al., 2020c). Older people feel restricted in engaging in functional activities. They also feel dissociated from socialization and are more concerned about restrictions on their social participation, such as being able to attend church, weddings, and visit friends (Awuviry-Newton et al., 2020c). Often, older men are more likely to experience a decrease in social networks compared to older women, because they are accused of abandoning their children when their children were young (Aboderin, 2004; Darkwa, 2000). Though older people in Ghana understand and admit to the functional restrictions they experience, these restrictions often lead to emotional and psychological instabilities such as anxiety, worry, and discomfort (Awuviry-Newton et al., 2020c). When older people become overwhelmed with stress, they feel unable to engage in social and other activities meant to enhance their health, which may lead to increasingly poor health, premature mortality, or suicide (Awuviry-Newton et al., 2020c).

One fascinating aspect of the functional disabilities older people experience is that they strive to be healthy and productive despite these difficulties (Awuviry-Newton et al., 2020c). Even amid their challenges, they want to be active. This desire highlights the need for caregivers or other people to support them by providing LTC at home. Having the ability to provide for the toileting difficulty care needs of older people is influenced by personal needs (such as advanced age), health, participation, and environmental factors. These factors include public and religious meeting attendance, socialization with co-workers, nearness to and availability of toilet facility, security, suffering from stroke and being a widow (Awuviry-Newton et al., 2019).

Another component of the holistic perspective influencing LTC is the physical and social environment. Currently, in Ghana, the built and social environments are not favourable for older people (Biritwum et al., 2013a), which seemingly add to the burdens of their lives. For example, poor roads and unreliable and inaccessible vehicles increase the care needs of older people in the country. The difficulty older people experience in accessing transport may limit their participation in activities they cherish and inhibit their ability to seek health care (Awuviry-Newton & Ofori-Dua, in press). Other environmental factors include the availability of caregivers for older people in Ghana, particularly looking at the absence of or few existing institutional care facilities, the lack of neighbourhood support, and older people reporting being misunderstood by friends and family (Awuviry-Newton et al., 2020d).

There are also personal factors that are intrinsic to the nature of older people that can make them more vulnerable to needing care. Broadly, an example of these individual factors includes demographic and socio-economic characteristics. Presently, in Ghana, evidence shows that many older people have a caregiver available to care for them; however, some older people are less likely to have one. Older people living as widows and having between two and four children are less likely to have a caregiver available (Awuviry-Newton, Nkansah, & Ofori-Dua, 2020a; Awuviry-Newton et al., 2020d). Additionally, older people living with a single health condition are less likely to have a caregiver available compared to older people living with multiple chronic conditions.

The intersection of the care needs of older people and caregivers' provision of care to older people enhances our understanding of caregiving's impact on both of these groups. In Ghana, caregivers' desire to commit themselves to care for older people was mainly influenced by reciprocity, despite the presence of internal and external stressors (Awuviry-Newton, Tavener, Wales, & Byles, in press).

That caregivers provide care to older people based on reciprocity draws attention to the fact that some older people in Ghana may experience neglect, exploitation, and abuse (Awuviry-Newton et al., 2020a). Older people face financial challenges, poor health, social isolation, lack of decent accommodation, nutritional food, and lack of choice over meals (Nkansah, Awuviry-Newton, Gyasi, Newton, & Boateng, 2021). Notably, older people who did not care for their children and those who did not have children would be most affected. Moreover, caregivers do not ignore their personal needs but are conscious of fulfilling them. The challenges and burdens caregivers incur could overwhelm the perceived benefits they receive (Awuviry-Newton et al., in press), which casts doubt on the sustainability of their care to older people living with functional difficulties in Ghana. Nowadays, many caregivers in Ghana do not express willingness to help older people meet their needs in terms of poor health and physical wellbeing (Awuviry-Newton et al., in press; Nortey, Aryeetey, Aikins, Amendah, & Nonvignon, 2017; Sanuade & Boatemaa, 2015).

When listening to older people describe their state of neglect, they attribute their deprivation of care and protection to death of partners, their failure to make the best decisions in the past, the failure of government institutions, and the breakdown of the extended family system (Awuviry-Newton et al., 2020a). For these older people, their care needs can be better understood from the amalgamation of these various, holistic factors.

2.2. Understanding the Needs of Caregivers

Generally, in sub-Saharan Africa, including Ghana, caregivers of older people are related by family and often report mixed experiences of caregiving. Just as in Botswana (Unanka, 2002), caregivers in Ghana often do not plan to become caretakers, but instead are relatively unprepared to assume the responsibility and change in their role. These abrupt responsibilities often require some sacrifices on the parts of the caregivers, who are motivated to accept the caregiving duty. For instance, caregivers of older people sacrifice by giving up their work, changing the nature of their job, or losing their job altogether to be able to provide for older people (Awuviry-Newton et al., in press; Van der Geest, 2002b). Awuviry-Newton et al. (in press) report that the sacrifices caregivers make is a manifestation of their level of commitment to satisfying the care needs of older people with whom they have established a caring relationship. Other motivations influencing the caregivers are reciprocity, an opportunity to obey God, setting an example for their children, taking it as a duty, the fear of social censure, or due to permissible conditions (Awuviry-Newton et al., in press). Moreover, caregivers report some benefits, such as exposure to learning new skills and knowledge for life, feeling happy, and receiving spiritual blessings (Awuviry-Newton et al., in press; Van der Geest, 2002b).

The overemphasis on fulfilling the needs of older people results in the compounding of the care burdens (Awuviry-Newton et al., in press). Caregivers report experiencing emotional, health, and physical burdens from caregiving (Awuviry-Newton et al., in press; Nortey et al., 2017; Sanuade & Boatemaa, 2015). According to Sanuade and Boatemaa (2015), less than 5% receive financial, emotional, health, physical and personal care support.

The negative experiences caregivers face, together with other predictors, often influence whether people will make themselves available to care for older people in Ghana. A recent study in the country reports the predictors of caregiver availability as i) older people advanced age, ii) being a widow, iii) living with a chronic condition, iv) hardly to be being understood by friends and family, v) having no neighbourhood support, and, vi) having two to four children (Awuviry-Newton et al., 2020d).

The negative consequences of these experiences often lead to inadequate and/or insufficient nature of LTC provision for older people (Awuviry-Newton et al., 2020a; Van der Geest, 2002b). Many older people report that caregivers provide insufficient material support (such as finances and food), irregular visitation by children and siblings, and in some cases adult children taking too long to respond to the needs of older people (Aboderin, 2004; Awuviry-Newton et al., 2020a).

3. The Evolution of Familial Care and Support for Older People In Ghana

3.1. Nature of Care in the Past

In Ghana, the extended family has long been the primary source of support for older people in times of illness and frailty (Apt, 1993, 1996; Awuviry-Newton, Byles, & Tavener, 2017; Kumado & Gockel, 2003; Ofori-Dua, 2014). Before colonization, life in Ghana was mainly rural with a patriarchal social system based on kinship (Ofori-Dua, 2014; Ray, 1986), with solidarity and mutual respect being the core features of the traditional Ghanaian way of life (Nyanguru, 2008; UNICEF, 2009). Extended family, an honoured institution, offered social and economic support to older people in times of economic hardship, disability, and isolation (Kumado & Gockel, 2003; Nukunya, 2003).

Kumado and Gockel (2003) emphasized the relevance of the extended family whereby "extended family practices transcended socio-economic protection to offering psychological stability and moral upliftment" (Kumado & Gockel, 2003, p. 1). In the past, older people imparted wisdom to the younger generation in Ghanaian society. This explains the reason why, when an older person dies, Ghanaians say "a library has caught fire" (Nyanguru, 2008, p. 52). Older people were respected in Ghanaian society because they were considered as seniors and the repository of socio-cultural customs and traditions (Van der Geest, 1997). However, the nature of care and support for older people has reportedly broken down (Brown, 1999; Nukunya, 2003; Ofori-Dua, 2014), with some reasons for this discussed in the next section.

3.2. Care and Support for Older People in Modern Ghana

Following the breakdown of family-based care for older people in Ghana (Awuviry-Newton et al., 2017), adult children (children aged 18+years) assumed the responsibility for the care of older people (Brown, 1999; Nortey et al., 2017; Nukunya, 2003; Ofori-Dua, 2014; Sackey, 2005; Sanuade & Boatemaa, 2015; Van der Geest, 2002b). The World Health Organization's Study on Global Ageing and Adult Health (SAGE) Ghana Wave 1 confirmed that adult children provide most of the care and support (91%) for older people (Biritwum, Mensah, Yawson, & Minicuci, 2013b).

Several factors have accounted for the breakdown of the traditional extended care and support for older people. One important factor explaining these changes is migration. For example, Van der Geest (2002b) reports how the movement of farmers to other rural areas—where they could acquire vast tracts of arable land—led to the separation of family members. Migration to urban centres or abroad has also accounted for the breakdown in traditional family ties (Brown, 1999; Nyanguru, 2008; Oppong, 2006). For instance, in the wake of the economic instability of the 1980s, when about two million Ghanaians left the country to work abroad, 63% of older people lost the support provided by one or more of their children (Government of Ghana, 2010).

Other factors for the described situation include the modernization of society, comprising changes such as the introduction of formal education, population growth, the establishment of a capitalist economy, economic hardship, and the arrival of numerous religious doctrines (Nukunya, 2003; Ofori-Dua, 2014; Van der Geest, 2002b). Education has led to the instilling of modern values, inquiring minds, and the projection of new models of social relations, which place more importance on independence over interdependence (Nyanguru, 2008). Similarly, the arrival of the Europeans in the 15th century brought Christianity to the land, which placed more focus on the nuclear family (Nukunya, 2003). For example, Ofori-Dua (2014) noted that during the Christian marriage ceremony, pastors refer to biblical scripts advising couples to leave their family and become a new one.

Another factor has to do with the introduction of the Intestate Succession Law (Government of Ghana, 1985), which allowed the immediate family of the deceased to take control of family properties (Ofori-Dua, 2014). Prior to the introduction of this law, for example, customs of the Akan ethnicity (the dominant ethnic group in Ghana) required that when a father died, his nephews were obliged to take control of the property and to take care of the entire family (Ofori-Dua, 2014). Currently, the widow is given the sole right to the family property to be used to take care of the children and other demands. This system has broken the interdependence and mutuality that brought together the extended family system and given way to the nucleated form of families in Ghana.

In summary, the literature has identified several factors behind the decline in traditional wider familial care and support for older people in Ghana, changing the pattern observed in traditional Ghana and leaving the burden of care on one's adult children (Brown, 1999; Nukunya, 2003). Other factors that have accounted for this change include the employment of women, modernization of society, rural-urban migration, and education. These changes are irreversible (Brown, 1999; Nukunya, 2003; Nyanguru, 2008; Ofori-Dua, 2014; Oppong, 2006; Van der Geest, 2002a). In a country where nursing homes, non-contributory social pensions and government support of aged caregivers are non-existent, adult children may not be able to care for older people, despite their best efforts (Van der Geest, 2002a, 2002b). Further research is needed to gain a more precise, in-depth understanding of the extent of the met and unmet needs and the best balance between formal and informal care for older people in Ghana.

4. RESPONDING TO AGEING IN GHANA

4.1. The Current State of Social and Health Services

Today, government programs aimed at reducing older people's vulnerability are mainly concerned with pensions and providing access to health care. These include the Livelihood Empowerment against Poverty (LEAP) (Government of Ghana, 2008), National Health Insurance Scheme (NHIS) (Government of Ghana, 2003), and Social Security and National Insurance Trust (Government of Ghana, 2009) programs (Table 1).

Table 1. Government social and health services

Social protection	Benefits	Beneficiaries	Institution in charge	Year
LEAP	Financial support	Orphans/ vulnerable children, people over 65 years and people with disabilities	Ministry of Gender, Children and Social Protection*	2008
NHIS	Basic healthcare services to residents through mutual and private health insurance schemes	All Ghanaians	Ministry of Health	2003
Social Security and National Insurance Trust	Financial insurance	Pensioners (60+years)	National Pension Regulatory Authority (NPRA)	2009

Source: Author's own.

* Formerly Ministry of Manpower, Youth and Employment.

With regards to LEAP, eligible older people aged 65 years and above living in extreme poverty without any form of support receive a grant from the Ministry of Gender, Children and Social Protection and are expected to enrol in the NHIS (Government of Ghana, 2007). The grants are minimal (between US$6 and US$12 bimonthly), so they are insufficient to cover the needs of older people living in dire poverty, many of whom also lack family support (Dako-Gyeke & Oduro, 2013; Gbedemah, Jones, & Pereznieto, 2010). In addition to the inadequacy of the grants, bureaucratic mismanagement has been found to delay cash payments to eligible beneficiaries (Abebrese, 2011).

The NHIS (Government of Ghana, 2003) is a social intervention that aims to ensure equitable health insurance for all Ghanaians, including older people (UNICEF, 2009). The NHIS covers prescriptions for diseases such as malaria, diarrhoea, upper respiratory tract infection, skin diseases, hypertension, diabetes and asthma (Government of Ghana, 2003).

Aside from this disease coverage, district-wide schemes are permitted under the law to cover many other diseases as much as possible, as long as the National Health Insurance Council approves them. Retired public servants, people aged 70 years and over, childless older people aged 60-69, pregnant women, children under 18 years of age, and the extremely poor are exempt from making premium payments for health care (Ministry of Health, 2015). Aside from these groups of people exempted from premium payment, every Ghanaian, including caregivers, pay a premium to enjoy the benefits of the NHIS. The NHIS allows the holder to receive basic healthcare without needing to make financial payment at the point of service delivery (Government of Ghana, 2003; Ministry of Health, 2015). Table 2 describes the contribution payable by the social groups in the informal sector (not working for the government).

Irrespective of these provisions, the NHIS does not cover the costs of treatment of chronic conditions, which are prevalent in old age (Kpessa-Whyte & Tsekpo, 2020). Examples of conditions that are not covered by the NHIS are optical aids, hearing aids, orthopaedic aids, dentures, beautification surgery, the supply of AIDS drugs, treatment of chronic kidney disease, heart and brain surgery (Government of Ghana, 2003).

In Ghana, there are no geriatric care units to care for the needs of older people (Ghana Business News, 2013). A study that assessed the country's policy and programs reported that Ghana has a healthcare system that, with a necessary boost, can address the health needs of older people (Araujo de Carvalho et al., 2015). As a result, the government has subsequently included additional measures to incorporate the health of older people into the health care system (Araujo de Carvalho et al., 2015).

Table 2. Contributions payable by the social groupings in the informal sector under the NHIS

Group		Description	Minimum contributions payable annually
Core poor	A	Adults who are unemployed and do not receive any identifiable or constant support from elsewhere for survival.	Free
Very Poor	B	Adults who are unemployed but receive identifiable and consistent financial support from sources of low income Adults who are employed but receive low returns for their efforts and are unable to meet their basic needs	GHc72,000 (USD1.22)
Middle income	D	Adults who are employed and able to meet their basic needs	GHc180,000 (USD3.06)
Rich	E	Adults who are able to meet their basic needs and some of their wants	GHc480,000 (USD8.15)
Very rich	F	Adults who are able to meet their needs and most of their wants	

Source: National Health Insurance Authority (2010).

In 2009, the government introduced a three-tiered pension policy, the Social Security and National Insurance Trust (SSNIT), to replace the previous Cap 30 plan (Government of Ghana, 2006, 2008). The Cap 30 was introduced in Ghana by the Pension Ordinance in 1946 by the British Colonial Government for Pensionable Officers in the Civil Service and members of the armed forces in the former British West African colonies. The scheme covered pensionable officers and African civil servants who joined the service before January 1972 (National Development Planning Commission, 2007). The newly introduced SSNIT comprises contributory social insurance and individual private pensions for the working population and voluntary contributions from those who work in businesses that are not controlled by the government (Kpessa, 2011b). However, workers in the informal sector are unable to contribute to long-term savings plans toward their income security in old age due to their limited income (Kpessa, 2011a, 2011b). Moreover, because the SSNIT is salary-based, it is difficult for informal sector workers, who constitute the majority of the working population, to amass insurance entitlements. Six years after its inception, only 7.6% of people aged 65 years and older received a pension under this scheme (HelpAge International, 2015).

While Ghana has no formal institutional care system or nursing homes for older people (Ofori-Dua, 2014; Van der Geest, 2002b), some non-governmental organizations provide care and support for older people. These include HelpAge International, Christian Health Association of Ghana, Sight Savers, Home Care Center, Ripples and Care for the Aged Foundation. These programs do not meet the needs of all older people and are facing increasing financial challenges due to the increasing ageing population (Van der Geest, 2016). For instance, the Care for Aged Foundation (formerly known as Akrowa Aged life foundation) provides a variety of individualized services for older people who do not have a family. The kinds of services provided include personal care such as bathing, grooming, dressing wounds, accompanying older people to hospital for an appointment and offering companionship (World Health Organisation, 2017). This organization began operation with 150 older people and as of 2017 had expanded its capacity to serve 400, with about 3000 older people on the waiting list (World Health Organisation, 2014).

4.2. The National Policy on Long-Term Care

Ghana introduced a National Ageing Policy in 2010 (Government of Ghana, 2010) aimed at promoting the health and overall well-being of older people in the country. At present Ghana has no specialized LTC policy for older people; however, the National Ageing Policy seems to ensure the continuation of LTC for older people by their families. Although the introduction of this policy shows a high level of commitment for improving the well-being of older people, the implementation of the various sub-policies have been problematic (World Health Organisation, 2014). The problems in moving the policy forward are the result of the lack of an implementation plan, which is needed for Ghanaian health services to carry out their duties. Moreover, there is a fair understanding of the policy among key senior health staff (World Health Organization, 2014). Other researchers have also criticized the country's policy for its lack of insight, stemming from the policymakers' shallow knowledge of the needs and insights of older people (Van der Geest, 2016).

The Ghana National Ageing Policy (GOG, 2010) was developed using the principles and priority areas of the Madrid International Plan of Action on Ageing and the African Union Policy Framework and Plan of Action on Ageing (Ghana National Country Assessment Report, 2013). The policy takes into consideration the health conditions that affect older people and their quest to live a healthy lifestyle. The policy further highlights the relevance of strengthening the support available to local communities to improve their health care delivery to older people, along with an expansion in palliative care serves and their integration into a comprehensive healthcare service for older people. It also states that adequate training and incentives will be provided to attract students to specialized training in geriatrics and gerontology (Government of Ghana, 2010). Further, the policy seeks to provide financial and healthcare resources to strengthen intergenerational family bonds, to enhance the availability of care and support for older people when they need it. The Ghana National Ageing Policy (Government of Ghana, 2010) shows that the government has some commitment to ensuring the well being of the growing older population. Although no program has been established in recent years in Ghana, the policy seeks to place more emphasis on the role of the traditional familial care and support for older people. Van der Geest (2016) considered the policy's over-reliance on family-based care for older people not to be feasible in achieving the LTC needs of older people, given demographic and economic changes and family values drifting away from traditional care, partly due to an increasing shift to the nuclear family (Aboderin, 2006).

A better balance of family and state responsibility (Aboderin, 2006, p. 164), is necessary to secure the well-being of older people and their caregivers. The Ghana National Ageing Policy (Government of Ghana, 2010) report does not make any provision for a government-funded pension, which could improve the lives of older people who worked in businesses not controlled by the government. Moreover, there was no provision for LTC for the frail, vulnerable older population without children and living with a disability (Van der Geest, 2016).

5. Implications for the Future of Long-Term Care for Older People in Ghana

Approaches to care, particularly LTC, need to be considered from a multifactorial perspective since older people require multifactorial interventions. This approach is fundamental in the Ghanaian context, so that older individuals, policy, and health and social services will not overly rely on family members to provide LTC services. From the available Ghanaian literature on care, older people' care needs are influenced by many factors, including personal factors such as being widowed, health-related factors such as living with at least one chronic condition, and environmental factors such as security and availability of social connections. Successful LTC for Ghanaians would mean that older people—as well as family caregivers—receive better healthcare, emotional, and financial support. LTC will also require a mechanism to enhance their functional capacity and involve variety and choice in the services available, ensuring they are designed for older people, to meet their health and/or personal care needs. Effective LTC signifies that older people can live in safety and remain independent for longer, even though they may still require assistance with daily activities and some care.

Given our current understanding of what continuing and durable care for older people in Ghana should be, the sustainability of LTC can only be achieved if care is not left to family members alone. Particularly, adult children left with the provision of care cannot meet the demands of their ageing parent(s). Providing care for older people in their home also does not excuse the State from delivering much-needed provisions, in terms of caregivers' health care, financial support, and respite care services.

Given this understanding, at the same time as the State promotes an ageing-in-place model of LTC for older people, they must continue to provide for the health and social care of both older people and their caregivers. Moreover, although older people may prefer to be cared for in their homes, the value of institutional care in Ghana cannot be overlooked (Manful, Asamoah, & Bediako, 2015). The ageing-in-place model, whereby individuals are provided with necessary health services and social support where they live (Wiles, Leibing, Guberman, Reeve, & Allen, 2012), can extend to aged care homes, with the State proving opportunities for older people to enter into institutional LTC if they do not have children, have experienced neglect, or have lost their caregivers to either illness or death. Moreover, because LTC is better when based on adherence to older people's preferences (Nkansah et al., 2021), they may choose to go into institutional care homes for their end-of-life care, which can be coordinated and authorized by the State.

Another aspect of the State intervention requires that the National Ageing Policy to be updated to accommodate the LTC needs of older people explicitly. Currently, the National Ageing Policy perpetuates the traditional familial model above other things and tries to keep it alive, whereas adopting and implementing a more holistic approach to care could improve the functional capacity and overall well-being of older people. A multi-sectoral approach, with a special focus on formal and community care services for all older people with or without family care, could enhance long-term well being. Moreover, support groups and respite care systems made up of trained caregivers should be introduced to aid caregivers who provide LTC for frail older people at home. There is also a need for more research on caregiving for older people in Ghana to provide relevant data to aid policy and service development.

There should be an implementation of a well-designed LTC system to coordinate approaches for older people, including raising awareness of the need for whole-person care and improving health workers' knowledge for dealing with older people's health needs. It should also include broadening the coverage of National Health Insurance Schemes and making hearing devices and eyeglasses available to older people (World Health Organisation, October 2013). It is recommended that to improve the healthcare of older people in Ghana, there should be minimal use of psychoactive medication and preference for environmental modifications such as exercise and rehabilitation (Dovie, 2019).

The growth in the number and the proportion of older people in Ghana requires thinking about older people's LTC needs as multifactorial and needing holistic intervention that includes the State, caregivers, older people themselves, environmental modifications, and consideration of health and social factors. It is recommended that the State should assume responsibility for adopting and sustaining the LTC approaches for older people through financing activities geared toward meeting the LTC needs of this group. The State can invite and be willing to sponsor private individuals with feasible intervention plans to secure older people's LTC needs in Ghana.

REFERENCES

Abebrese, J. (2011). Social Protection in Ghana: An overview of existing programmes and their prospects and challenges. *Fredrich Ebert Stiftung, Germany*.

Aboderin, I. (2004). Decline Material Family Support for Older People in Urban Ghana, Africa: Understanding Processes and Causes of Change. *Gerontology: Social Sciences, 59B*(3), S128-S137.

Aboderin, I. (2006). *Intergenerational support and old age in Africa*: Transaction Publishers.

Amosun, S., Nyante, G., & Wiredu, E. (2013). Perceived and experienced restrictions in participation and autonomy among adult survivors of stroke in Ghana. *African Health Sciences, 13*(1), 24-31.

Apt, N. A. (1993). Care of the elderly in Ghana: An emerging issue. *Journal of Cross-Cultural Gerontology, 8*(4), 301-312.

Apt, N. A. (1996). *Coping with old age in a changing Africa. Social change and the elderly Ghanaian*. Aldershot, UK: Aveburg.

Araujo de Carvalho, I., Byles, J., Aquah, C., Amofah, G., Biritwum, R., Panisset, U., . . . Beard, J. (2015). Informing evidence-based policies for ageing and health in Ghana. *Bulletin of the World Health Organization, 93*(1), 47-51. doi:10.2471/BLT.14.136242

Awuviry-Newton, K., Byles, J., & Tavener, M. (2017). *Evolution of familial care and support for older people in Ghana: A literature review.* Paper presented at the Maintaining a work-life balance as a researcher, Western Australia.

Awuviry-Newton, K., Nkansah, J. O., & Ofori-Dua, K. (2020a). Attributions of elder neglect: A phenomenological study of older people in Ghana. *Health & Social Care in the Community, 28*(6), 2172-2178. doi:10.1111/hsc.13028.

Awuviry-Newton, K., & Ofori-Dua, K. (in press). Understanding Transportation difficulty among older adults in Ghana from the perspective of World Health Organisation's (WHO) Healthy Ageing framework: Lessons for Improving Social Work Practice with Older Adults. *British Journal of Social Work.*

Awuviry-Newton, K., Ofori-Dua, K., & Newton, A. (2020b). Correlates of older adult inpatients' personal care provision to people with functional difficulties in Ghana. *PloS One, 15*(10), e0238693.

Awuviry-Newton, K., Tavener, M., Wales, K., & Byles, J. (2020c). Interpretative Phenomenological Analysis of the Lived Experiences of Older Adults Regarding Their Functional Activities in Ghana. *Journal of Primary Care & Community Health, 11.* doi:10.1177/2150132720931110.

Awuviry-Newton, K., Tavener, M., Wales, K., & Byles, J. (in press). Using Ethics of Care to understanding the lived experiences of caregivers providing care for older adults living with functional difficulties. *Journal of Ageing Studies.*

Awuviry-Newton, K., Tavener, M., Wales, K., Kowal, P., & Byles, J. (2019). Activities of daily living difficulties and toileting among older Ghanaians: an application of the WHO-ICF framework. *Innovation in Aging, 3*(Supplement_1), S520-S520.

Awuviry-Newton, K., Wales, K., Tavener, M., & Byles, J. (2020d). Do factors across the World Health Organisation's International Classification of Functioning, Disability and Health framework relate to caregiver availability for community-dwelling older adults in Ghana? *PloS One, 15*(5), e0233541.

Biritwum, R., Minicuci, N., Yawson, A., Theou, O., Mensah, G., Naidoo, N., . . . Jiang, Y. (2016). Prevalence of and factors associated with frailty and disability in older adults from China, Ghana, India, Mexico, Russia and South Africa. *Maturitas, 91*, 8-18.

Biritwum, R. B., Mensah, G., Minicuci, N., Yawson, A. E., Naidoo, N., Chatterji, S., & Kowal, P. (2013a). Household characteristics for older adults and study background from SAGE Ghana Wave 1. *Global Health Action, 6*(1), 20096.

Biritwum, R. B., Mensah, G., Yawson, A. E., & Minicuci, N. (2013b). Study on global AGEing and adult health (SAGE), Wave 1: the Ghana national report. *Geneva: World Health Organization.*

Brown, C. K. (1999). *Caring for the elderly: perspectives from Ghana and Japan*. Cape Coast: Catholic Mission Press.

Calys-Tagoe, B., Hewlett, S. A., Dako-Gyeke, P., Yawson, A. E., Bad-Doo, N. A., Seneadza, N. A. H., . . . Chatterji, S. (2014). Predictors of subjective well-being among older Ghanaians. *Ghana Medical Journal, 48*(4), 178-184.

Dako-Gyeke, M., & Oduro, R. (2013). Effects of houshold size on cash transfer utilization for ophans and vulnerable children in rural Ghana. *Academic Journal of Interdisciplinary Studies* (2), 239-251.

Darkwa, O. K. (2000). Toward a comprehensive understanding of the needs of elderly Ghanaians. *Ageing International, 25*(4), 65-79.

Debpuur, C., Welaga, P., Wak, G., & Hodgson, A. (2010). Self-reported health and functional limitations among older people in the Kassena-Nankana District, Ghana. *Global Health Action, 3*, 54-63. doi:10.3402/gha.v3i0.2151.

Dovie, D. A. (2019). The status of older adult care in contemporary Ghana: A profile of some emerging issues. *Frontiers in Sociology, 4*, 25.

Gbedemah, C., Jones, N., & Pereznieto, P. (2010). Gendered risks, poverty and vulnerability in Ghana: Is the LEAP cash transfer programme making a difference. *London: Overseas Development Institute.*

Ghana Business News. (2013). NHIS neglecting health needs of older people – HelpAge Ghana. Retrieved from https://www.ghanabusiness news.com/2013/04/19/nhis-neglecting-health-needs-of-older-people-helpage-ghana/.

Government of Ghana. (1985). *Memorandum to the Intestate Succession PNDC Law 111 of Ghana.*

Government of Ghana. (2003). National Health Insurance Scheme (NHIS). Retrieved 20th June, 2017, from Ministry of Gender, Children and Social Protection & Ministry of Health http://mogcsp.gov.gh /projects/ghana-national-household-registry-gnhr/.

Government of Ghana. (2006). *Presidential Commission on Pensions. Accra, Ghana*. Ghana.

Government of Ghana. (2007). *The national social protection strategy: Investing in people*. Accra.

Government of Ghana. (2008). *The National Pension Reform Bill*. Accra, Ghana.

Government of Ghana. (2009). Social Security and National InsuranceTrust (SSNIT). Retrieved 20/06/2017, from International Labour Organisation http://www.ilo.org/dyn/ilossi/ssimain.viewScheme?p_lang=en&p_scheme_id=129&p_geoaid=288.

Government of Ghana. (2010). *National Ageing Policy: Ageing with Security and Dignity*. Retrieved from.

He, W., Goodkind, D., & Kowal, P. R. (2016). *An aging world: 2015*: United States Census Bureau.

HelpAge International. (2015). *Global AgeWatch Index 2015*. Retrieved 16 January, 2017 http://www.helpage.org/global-agewatch/population-ageing-data/country-ageing-data/?country=Ghana.

Kpessa-Whyte, M., & Tsekpo, K. (2020). Lived Experiences of the Elderly in Ghana: Analysis of Ageing Policies and Options for Reform. *Journal of Cross-Cultural Gerontology*, 1-12.

Kpessa, M. W. (2011a). The politics of public policy in Ghana: From closed circuit bureaucrats to citizenry engagement. *Journal of Developing Societies, 27*(1), 29-56.

Kpessa, M. W. (2011b). Retirement income security under Ghana's three-tier pension model: Assessment of risks and options for reform. *Pensions: An International Journal, 16*(2), 127-136. doi:10.1057/pm.2011.10.

Kumado, K., & Gockel, A. F. (2003). *A study on social security in Ghana.* Accra: Friedrich Ebert Stiftung.

Manful, E., Asamoah, E., & Bediako, A. B. (2015). Care in the Silver Years: Academics Perception of Institutional Care for the Elderly in Ghana. *Mediterranean Journal of Social Sciences*. doi:10.5901/mjss.2015.v6n6s4p220.

Ministry of Health. (2015). *Holistic assessment of the health sector program of work 2014*. Accra.

National Health Insurance Authority. (2010). National Health Insurance Scheme annual report. In: Author Accra, Ghana.

Nkansah, O. J., Awuviry-Newton, K., Gyasi, M., Newton, A., & Boateng, A. S.-A. (2021). "Who doesn't Have Challenges? I Have a Lot of Challenges": Exploring the Challenges and Coping Strategies of Neglected Older Adults in Ghana. *Journal of Cross-Cultural Gerontology*. doi:10.1007/s10823-020-09419-3.

Nortey, S. T., Aryeetey, G. C., Aikins, M., Amendah, D., & Nonvignon, J. (2017). Economic burden of family caregiving for elderly population in southern Ghana: the case of a peri-urban district. *International Journal For Equity In Health, 16*(1), 16.

Nukunya, G. K. (2003). *Tradition and Change in Ghana: An Introduction to Sociology*. Accra: University Press.

Nyanguru, A. C. (2008). Aging and the elderly in the family: A changing African Scenario. In *Changing family systems: A global perspective.* (Tapogo M., Levers, L. L. & Jacques, G., (Eds.) ed.). Botswana: Bay Publishing, Gaborone.

Ofori-Dua, K. (2014). *Extended Family Support and Elderly Care in Bamang, Ashanti Region of Ghana.* (PhD). University of Ghana.

Oppong, C. (2006). Familial roles and social transformations: Older men and women in sub-Saharan Africa. *Research on Aging, 28*(6), 654-668.

Orji, B. C., Rao, N., Thompson, E., & Brieger, W. R. (2017). Community health workers provide integrated community case management using malaria rapid diagnostic test kits. *Research in Social and Administrative Pharmacy, 13*(4), 875-879.

Peltzer, K., Hewlett, S., Yawson, A., Moynihan, P., Preet, R., Wu, F., . . . Chatterji, S. (2014). Prevalence of loss of all teeth (edentulism) and associated factors in older adults in China, Ghana, India, Mexico, Russia and South Africa. *International Journal of Environmental Research and Public Health, 11*(11), 11308-11324.

Ray, D. I. (1986). *Ghana: politics, economics and society*. Burns & Oates.

Sackey, H. A. (2005). *Female labour force participation in Ghana: The effects of education.*

Sanuade, O. A., & Boatemaa, S. (2015). Caregiver profiles and determinants of caregiving burden in Ghana. *Public Health, 129*(7), 941-947.

Unanka, G. O. (2002). Family support and health status of the elderly in Imo State of Nigeria. *Journal of Social Issues, 58*(4), 681-695.

UNICEF. (2009). *Social protection and children: Opportunities and challenges in Ghana*. Accra

United Nations. (2017). *World population prospects: The 2017 Revision Volume I: Comprehensive Tables*. Retrieved from New York.

United Nations, Department of Economic and Social Affairs, & Division, P. (2019a). *World Population Prospects 2019*. Retrieved from.

United Nations, Department of Economic and Social Affairs, & Division, P. (2019b). *World Population Prospects 2019: Highlights*. Retrieved from https://www.google.com/url?sa=t&rct=j&q=&esrc=s&source=web&cd=&cad=rja&uact=8&ved=2ahUKEwjz64uSnZ_sAhVozjgGHa8mBC4QFjAAegQIAxAC&url=https%3A%2F%2Fpopulation.un.org%2Fwpp%2FPublications%2FFiles%2FWPP2019_Highlights.pdf&usg=AOvVaw1VFJah-iC4isgp8DJHVa_o.

Van der Geest, S. (1997). Money and Respect: The Changing Value of Old Age in Rural Ghana. *Africa* (4), 64.

Van der Geest, S. (2002a). From Wisdom to Witchcraft: Ambivalence Towards Old Age in Rural Ghana. *Africa* (3), 72.

Van der Geest, S. (2002b). Respect and reciprocity: Care of elderly people in rural Ghana. *Cross-Cultural Gerontology, 17*, 3-31.

Van der Geest, S. (2016). Will families in Ghana continue to care for older people? Logic and contradiction in policy. In *Ageing in Sub-Saharan Africa: Spaces and Practices of Care* (pp. 21-41). London: Policy Press.

Wiles, J. L., Leibing, A., Guberman, N., Reeve, J., & Allen, R. E. (2012). The meaning of "aging in place" to older people. *The Gerontologist, 52*(3), 357-366.

World Health Organisation. (2014). *Ghana country assessment report on ageing and health.* Retrieved 5 January, 2017 http://apps.who.int/iris/bitstream/10665/126341/1/9789241507332_eng.pdf.

World Health Organisation. (2017). *Towards long-term care systems in sub-Saharan Africa: WHO series on long-term care*. Retrieved from Geneva: https://www.who.int/ageing/long-term-care/en/.

World Health Organisation. (October 2013). *Ghana: looking after its older people.* Retrieved from https://www.who.int/features/2013/ghana-living-longer/en/.

In: The Future of Long-Term Care
Editor: Pablo Villalobos Dintrans
ISBN: 978-1-53619-263-6

Chapter 5

ADDRESSING LONG-TERM CARE FINANCING CHALLENGES IN THE UNITED ARAB EMIRATES

Ahmed Saleh Al Awlaqi*
Paris-Sorbonne University Abu Dhabi,
Abu Dhabi, United Arab Emirates

ABSTRACT

Long-term care financing continues to be a major challenge in the United Arab Emirates, as the bulk of the existing financial budget allocation is largely committed to meeting primary and secondary healthcare needs. The objective of this chapter is to examine the potential challenges that continue to define long-term care needs in the United Arab Emirates. A critical assessment of previously published literature in the chapter identifies several challenges that need to be addressed to improve the state of long-term care services in the United Arab Emirates. Results reveal that the current financial resources committed to long-term care services fail to meet the needs of patients, prompting the need for travel overseas for medical treatment. Lack of a regulatory body committed to long-term care needs implies that the sector is not

* Corresponding Author's E-mail: uaemarati2030@gmail.com.

prioritized, as it is considered part of the general healthcare system. As a result, there is often poor long-term service delivery as patients seek high-cost home care and nursing services to access essential care for chronic medical conditions. Due to limited allocation of financial and other resources, there is often a shortage of personnel, such as specialist doctors and nurses, which is further compounded by the shortage of hospital beds. Thus, there is a need for urgent healthcare financing reforms to ensure dedicated facilities and resources are available to address long-term care needs in the United Arab Emirates.

1. Introduction

In the last two decades, the United Arab Emirates (UAE) has experienced substantial economic growth resulting in a high human development index in education, life expectancy, and per capita income. As a result of improved economic status, there have been growing concerns about lifestyle change, dietary consumption, and changing healthcare needs. Abduelkarem et al. (2020) noted that the changing socio-economic status has contributed to growing cases of obesity, diabetes, kidney disease, and other lifestyle diseases among the younger population. A cross-sectional study by AlKetbi, Grivna, and Al Dhaheri (2020) revealed a high rate of depression, distraction, and psychological problems among young people who engage in reckless driving, resulting in chronic injuries and permanent disabilities. Alao et al., (2020) further reported increased numbers of people requiring chronic assistance with daily living due to falls, occupational hazards, and trauma. The relatively long-life expectancy of 78 years in the UAE implies that older generations require support with care for chronic conditions such as heart disease, diabetes, intensive care support, and mental health services, further straining the limited healthcare resources (Gachiri, 2017). Malik et al., (2020) noted that most of the patients with chronic care needs have low compliance with medications and going for clinical appointments, thereby requiring close care support. The World Health Organization (WHO) reports that a third of adults in the UAE are obese, and one out of five people live with diabetes. As the incidence of lifestyle diseases increases, these populations, supported by relatively high levels of income, will demand higher quality healthcare (WHO, 2020). The government's focus is on developing a healthcare infrastructure to address this demand (Export.gov., 2020).

Underwriting the above considerations, there is a need to have robust mechanisms to address potential challenges among Emiratis with various chronic conditions. Long-term care (LTC) has been a fundamental approach to meeting the needs of individuals who require close support and assisted living (Nadash, Doty, & von Schwanenflügel, 2017). Pozo-Rubio, Pardo-García, and Escribano-Sotos (2020) shared that adequate planning in terms of resource allocation to LTC services has critical implications for the sustainability of chronic care services and assisted living in the UAE. According to Fasseeh et al., (2020), increasing the allocation in the public budget and enhanced institutionalization are critical factors in the implementation of LTC services. With the increasingly aging population and weakening traditional family ties that would require younger generations to care for older people, there is a growing need to improve service delivery within LTC facilities in the UAE and across the Gulf region (Gaili et al., 2019). To address this rising demand, some Gulf nations such as Saudi Arabia, Oman, and the UAE have launched a series of policy initiatives aimed at developing a robust LTC system in collaboration with the private sector (Paulo, 2019). Although current policies focus on boosting supply and building infrastructure for service provision, financing the recurrent cost of LTC services and making them widely affordable is a key challenge in the UAE. LTC services are expensive and have been regarded as unsustainable (in terms of attracting private service providers) unless there is some dependable way of paying for them (Abu-Saad et al., 2019; Foster et al., 2019).

The purpose of this chapter is to review existing LTC financing systems in the Gulf region, with a specific focus on the UAE. The specific interest of this analysis is on examining key LTC financing challenges and resource allocation options for policymakers in the UAE in the wake of coronavirus disease of 2019 (COVID-19). Although still in its nascent stages, available data reveals that the COVID-19 pandemic has exposed many flaws in LTC financing, including barriers facing vulnerable patients for access and utilization of LTC services (Lehnert et al., 2019). Drawing on LTC financing insights gained from other parts of the world, such as the United States of America, Europe, and Asia, this chapter discusses potential implications of international experiences for UAE LTC services.

2. LTC Systems and Financing Options

LTC financing differs by country, and there is no uniform financing model. However, Moonesar, Elshokamy, and Sayani (2018) noted that when deliberating on LTC financing, policymakers typically consider the options of private and public financing to determine the model of funding, regulation, and resource allocation. Public funding for LTC services includes considering options such as universal coverage vs. means-test eligibility, and third-party payer or insurer vs. direct payer (Moonesar, Elshokamy, & Sayani, 2018). Some countries use universal coverage systems, while others use means-tested funding or combine both systems into a hybrid model (Garrow, 2020; Johnson & Wiener 2016).

Under means-tested funding, the main focus is to allocate benefits to poor individuals who are unable to afford to finance their care due to the high costs of medical bills (Campbell, 2014). The philosophical premise behind means-tested funding is that the government has a primary mandate to ensure medical access to younger and older people who have disabilities or are unable to provide for themselves. The means-tested funding system is being used in countries like the United States, New Zealand, and England (Nadash et al., 2017). However, in the UAE, means-tested funding has been largely limited to mainstream healthcare financing through the Thiqa scheme for UAE nationals and Basic and Enhanced schemes for expatriates (Moonesar, Elshokamy, & Sayani, 2018). In LTC financing, most funding comes from out-of-pocket payment by affected individuals who mostly seek private nursing services or home care services due to limited financial support by the government (Moonesar, Elshokamy, & Sayani, 2018).

By contrast, the universal coverage system is applied where social solidarity is highly valued and the right to LTC access is perceived in a similar manner as the right to medical care. Countries like Sweden, the Netherlands, France, Japan, and Germany use this funding system (Albarrán et al., 2019; Nadash et al., 2017). In Germany, the universal social insurance system for LTC is used as a primary source of funding for the LTC system, with a specific focus on home care and nursing homes for people of all ages with disabilities (Barczyk & Kredler, 2019). In Korea, the national LTC funding introduced in 2015 focuses on providing universal coverage for persons over 65 years old, regardless of income. As a joint funding program, the Korean LTC model is funded from out-of-pocket payments (15-20%), government subsidies (20%), and participants (60-65%) (Jung et al., 2014; Kwon 2009). Besides supporting older persons over 65 years, the program also supports individuals over 40 years with aging-related conditions such as Alzheimer's diseases and dementia. China and Taiwan have also developed a government-led LTC insurance through the universal coverage system (Yeh, 2019).

A second funding option includes the direct provision of LTC services that have also been used as an alternative to LTC funding; services are provided by non-governmental or government-run organizations. For example, in Sweden and other Scandinavian countries, most LTC providers are government institutions and agencies, although some efforts have been made towards privatization (Lindström et al., 2019; Meinow et al., 2020). Government provision of LTC services is based on increasing care delivery, irrespective of whether LTC services are profitable. Nonetheless, Meinow et al., (2020) shared that there is no arms-length association between payers and providers where government agencies are involved, resulting in a potential decline in spending efficiency. Service efficiency is achieved through third-party funding systems to finance healthcare through the private sector. The privatization approach to LTC funding is based on the assumption that competing organizations will provide multiple options to consumers, thereby resulting in flexibility in access, focusing on consumer needs, and lowering costs to customers. Third-party funding systems focus on enrolling eligible providers, determining eligible users, developing reimbursement rates, paying providers for services, and monitoring quality compliance.

The third funding consideration is based on examining the extent of government responsibility in healthcare financing and LTC service delivery. In countries such as Canada, the Netherlands, Sweden, and the United Kingdom, governments largely rely on subnational administrators to develop and administer their LTC systems. In Sweden, all responsibility for administering, financing, and organizing LTC services is delegated to municipalities, although Sweden is a small country with less than 10 million people (Lindström et al., 2019). Devolving LTC needs to local entities is based on three main postulations. One, municipalities, states, and provinces are heavily involved in many social services in most countries. Therefore, establishing a local approach to LTC services is key to creating an important link between chronic care and other LTC services, such as care for individuals with disabilities (Kümpel, & Schneider, 2020). Two, LTC is an intensely personal service that involves making choices about how medical users want to live their lives. Three, since subnational governments are less likely to routinize their decision-making processes and since their cases loom larger in the policy process, locally administered LTC programs are less likely to be bureaucratic and rigid compared to centrally managed programs (Kümpel, & Schneider, 2020).

Different from the devolved LTC system is the centralized and nationalized approach to LTC financing and service delivery. Key countries that use this approach include Japan and Germany. However, in some cases, governmental and subnational entities are still used to facilitate the same goal of optimal care delivery in terms of LTC financing and service access (Kümpel, & Schneider, 2020). For example, under the Japanese LTC insurance program, there are a total of 2,897 municipal governments or allied systems of municipalities that insure LTC services and have a primary mandate of providing optimal long-term chronic care services (Campbell, 2014). Nonetheless, considering that almost all aspects of LTC financing (such as reimbursement rates, most benefits, and eligibility) are fixed at the national level, municipalities are largely limited in shaping the funding and type of LTC services they provide. Therefore, even if premiums are set at the municipal level, almost all the parameters related to LTC financing are set at the national level. Service consolidation at the national level is based on two premises: one, that a uniform national program serves to guarantee horizontal equity across diverse geographical locations (Lorenz-Dant, 2020); two, that having in place a single national program may result in fewer service administration costs and other expenses because program systems and rules need to be created only once. At the same time, subnational units develop systems and procedures (Lehnert et al., 2019).

Besides public financing, the private sector also plays a key role in LTC financing, although private LTC insurance does not play a major role in financing LTC in any country (Arsenijevic et al., 2016). In France, which has significant market penetration, LTC insurance is integrated with health insurance, but the benefits are limited, and private insurance accounts for less than 1 percent of LTC expenditures. In Germany, private insurance is primarily offered for upper-income people and government officials as an alternative to the mandatory statutory sickness funds. In the United States, which has had an active market of private LTC insurance since the mid-1980s, only about 12% the 65-and-older population has any LTC insurance (almost all of which has substantial restrictions on coverage), and it accounts for only about 7 percent of total expenditures (Favreault et al., 2015).

In countries with LTC insurance, such as Germany, private LTC insurance may play a role in supplementing the public budget. In countries with means-tested financing systems, insurance is meant to substitute for government programs. However, there is often low market demand for private LTC insurance, for various reasons. Some of the potential reasons include: the fact that most people do not expect to need LTC insurance; medical underwriting excludes substantial numbers of people from purchasing policies; and the cost of private LTC insurance is high. An alternative approach to expanding the market would be for the government to pay for LTC costs beyond what is covered in an approved private LTC insurance policy. Such a strategy may be based on providing lifetime coverage without requiring people to buy a costly private LTC insurance policy that provides lifetime benefits, a type of policy that has largely disappeared from the marketplace.

Out-of-pocket spending is another part of private LTC financing, although it is not the principal source of financing in any country with a developed LTC service system. In countries with public LTC insurance, consumers typically must pay coinsurance for services or supplement the amount paid by the insurance plan (Orlovic et al., 2017). In Japan, there is a 10% coinsurance for services, except for the low-income population (Pozo-Rubio et al., 2020). The coinsurance has two purposes: (1) for home- and community-based services, coinsurance serves to limit demand for services that may be inherently desirable even to people who are not disabled, such as homemaker services, and (2) for institutional services, the co-payment amount is conceptually designed to be equivalent to the normal living costs of room and board that individuals would incur even if they were not disabled and living in a nursing home. In countries with public LTC insurance, such as Germany and Japan, means-tested public assistance programs provide help with the coinsurance for people who cannot afford it (Del Pozo-Rubio & Jiménez-Rubio, 2019).

3. Current Situation in the UAE

As of 2019, the estimated population size in the UAE was approximately 9.4 million people, out of which 85% are expatriates. At a natural increase of 1.3% per year, the UAE population doubles every 14 years (HAAD, 2017; Export.gov, 2020). Despite the potential structural deficit in human resources, delivery, and healthcare infrastructure, the UAE has largely developed a healthcare system focused on catering to the healthcare needs of its rapidly growing population.

Based on the Organization for Economic Cooperation and Development (OECD) standards, the availability of healthcare resources in the UAE is considered below average. Despite the number of physicians increasing substantially in the last two decades, reaching 27 doctors per 10,000 people, it remains below the OECD average of 32 physicians

(WHO, 2015; WHO, 2020). Moreover, by 2019 there were 56 nurses per 10,000 people in the UAE, much less than the average of 87 nurses in OECD countries (Tuite et al., 2020). The total hospital bed capacity in 2019 was 13,315 beds, which is an equivalent of 19 beds per 10,000 persons, below the average of 48 beds in OECD countries. By 2030, the Department of Health of Abu Dhabi projects the number of physicians to increase by 50% to cope with the needs of the UAE population and rising cases of chronic conditions (UAE Government, 2020).

According to a 2018 report released by the Health Authority of Abu Dhabi (HAAD), there is a growing problem in the imbalance between the supply of medical consultants and specialists in the seven Emiratis (HAAD, 2018). As a result of this shortage in healthcare providers, the LTC sector continues to experience an undersupply of specialists, with most providers being absorbed into primary healthcare facilities. In the last two years, however, there was an oversupply of medical providers in some specialties such as gynecology and medicine, especially in government facilities (HAAD, 2018). By contrast, there continues to be an undersupply of physicians in LTC-related services, such as chronic injury and trauma, substance abuse such as alcohol and other drugs, and oncology (Tuite et al., 2020). In addition to the shortage of personnel in LTC facilities, there are also increased concerns about funding challenges in other LTC fields such as pediatric surgery, rheumatology, and trauma and accidents. According to the Department of Health (2019), the undersupply of LTC specialist providers ranges from 0% to 60%. Considering the growing demand for chronic care experts in the wake of the COVID-19 pandemic (Tuite et al., 2020), one may only anticipate that the LTC sector will be strained in delivering optimal care to patients in coming years.

An additional challenge reported in the UAE healthcare system is the growing overreliance on expatriate medical personnel (Lapão, 2018; WHO 2019). For instance, in Abu Dhabi, an estimated 82% of the residents are non-nationals, with up to 96% of the healthcare workers being expatriates. By contrast, the Dubai Statistics Centre estimates that 91% of the population in Dubai are expatriates, where 90% of the healthcare personnel are non-locals (Dubai Health Authority, 2017). As such, the large proportion of expatriate employees within the healthcare industry presents a challenge to LTC human resource management due to the high turnover rate among expatriate employees (WHO, 2019; WHO, 2020). AlQutob et al., (2020) reported that high voluntary turnover rates among healthcare workers contribute to delays in LTC delivery due to challenges with replacing skilled professionals in different specialties and sub-specialties. These statistics reveal that when assessing the current state of LTC services in the UAE, there are potential concerns about uncertainty in human resources, especially in developing local human resource capacity to meet the rising demand for LTC services.

Infrastructure challenges also compound the problems experienced in the UAE LTC sector. The UAE Government (2020) has reported efforts to renovate existing medical facilities and construct new hospitals based on private and public financing. A key focus of this partnership is to close the growing gap in the number of hospital beds by 2025 by installing facilities to meet the current deficit of about 8,000 beds, thereby encouraging private sector investment. As of 2019, the government reported a shortage of up to 2,000 beds across the UAE, despite a 30% increase in the number of hospital beds in the last decade. Compared to other Gulf Cooperation Council (GCC) countries, the UAE has the lowest hospital bed capacity of 1.4 hospital beds per 1,000 residents, compared with the regional average of 4.3 hospital beds per 1,000 residents. The disparity is worse when considering the LTC sector, where the UAE has 0.6 hospital beds per 1000 residents compared to the regional average of 5.8 hospital beds per 1,000 residents (AlQutob et al., 2020). There are also growing concerns that limited training opportunities for local populations continue to exacerbate the burden of delivering optimal care to residents across the seven Emiratis (Export.gov., 2020). With the growing medical tourism sector, there is a need for increased funding and financing of more hospital beds to meet the needs of both local and international patients (Export.gov., 2020).

The key challenges within the UAE healthcare sector are addressed by the Ministry of Health (MOH), which is tasked with representing the federal government, and the Dubai Health Authority (DHA), which represents the local government in Dubai. In contrast, HAAD represents the local government in Abu Dhabi. Health services are delivered by private facilities, DHA, and MOH, including the Dubai Healthcare City (DHCC). The DHA owns twenty-four hospital facilities with a capacity of 2,063 beds, in addition to 14 primary healthcare facilities (PHCs). By contrast, the MOH has two hospital facilities with a capacity of 287 beds, with nine PHCs in Dubai. The private sector has an estimated 22 hospitals with a bed capacity of 1,468 beds and over 1,200 polyclinics and outpatient clinics. The Joint Commission International (JCI) has accredited about 95% of the hospitals in DHA. Despite the existing hospital bed capacity and facility accreditation, most of the resources are limited to supporting primary and secondary healthcare needs in the UAE, with few financial resources allocated to meet tertiary needs of local residents, such as LTC.

3.1. General Healthcare Financing

Total health expenditures (THE), which consist of current health expenditures (CHE) and capital formation, are no longer included in the National health accounts (NHAs). This was decided based on recommendations from the System of Health Accounts (SHA) 2011, and CHE is included instead. The CHE includes all expenses on health services, but excludes investments and exports (Favreault et al., 2015; Lehnert et al., 2019). THE in the UAE was 10.8 billion United Arab Emirates Dirham (AED) in 2012, equivalent to 3.4% of gross domestic product. This is more than 6 percentage points lower than the OECD average of 9.3% (Lord et al., 2018; Unroe et al., 2017). The CHE constituted about 92% of THE, equivalent to 9.9 billion AED, and capital formation constitutes about 8%, equivalent to 867 million AED. By 2019, there were four main healthcare financing schemes in the UAE (Pearson et al., 2019).

- The federal and local governments funded 33% of CHE and pooled 38% of CHE via local and governmental schemes;

- Employers funded and pooled 36% of CHE via private health insurance;
- Households funded and pooled about 22% of CHE; and
- Corporations funded about 9% of CHE and pooled about 4% of CHE via enterprise financing schemes.

The UAE Government allocates a significant share of the federal budget for the healthcare sector every year to provide quality medical services. However, the LTC sector receives less than 2% of total healthcare financing, further indicating the resource strain within the LTC sector (Pearson et al., 2019). Figure 1 presents the financial allocation by the UAE government to the healthcare sector for the years 2016-2020, based on the draft budgets for those years (UAE Government, 2020).

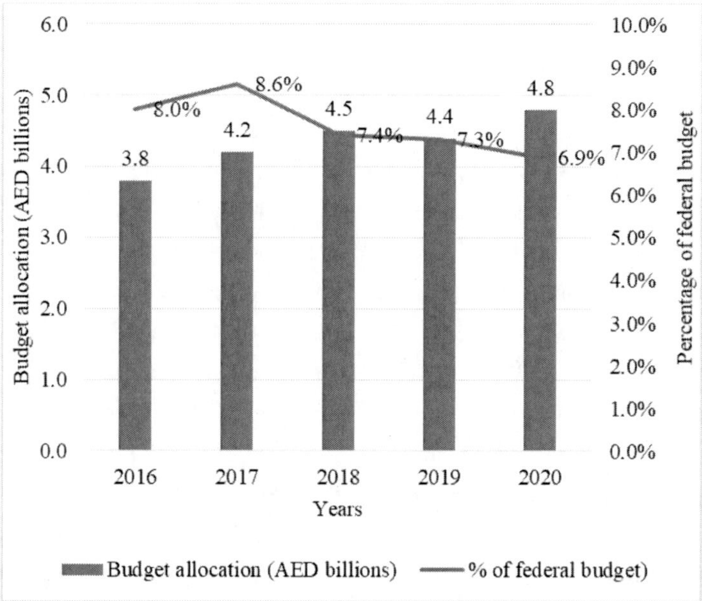

Source: UAE Government (2020).

Figure 1. UAE healthcare financing between 2016 and 2020.

In all cases, there is a mandatory health insurance model that funds the national healthcare system in the UAE. Key additional funding sources for the healthcare sector in the UAE include:

- Sponsors or Employers Funding: All UAE employers are responsible for providing their workers or employees with health insurance. Individuals who are not employed, however, must be insured through their respective sponsors.
- Government Funding: The UAE government is a single-payer health system for all Emirati nationals, and it is administered by the national health insurance company, which is regulated by the Ministry of Health and Prevention (MOHAP).
- Individual Funding: Healthcare financing is also achieved through out-of-pocket payments in addition to premiums paid to health insurance firms.

In the UAE, healthcare funding regulation is undertaken at the Emirati and the Federal level. Federal funding legislation dates back to the 1970-1980s, and there are continuous reforms focused on facilitating competitive healthcare development. However, existing literature lacks specific insight on how the UAE regulates LTC financing and/or the delivery of LTC care. In efforts to address LTC financing needs and resource allocation, the UAE government has been actively liberalizing the healthcare sector in attempts aimed at attracting foreign investments, with a specific focus on improving the financing of LTC sector and boosting access to LTC facilities (Export.gov, 2020). As of 2019, THE in the UAE was valued at AED 14.8 billion. This figure includes healthcare expenditures from all seven Emirates, in addition to their funding contributions to the federal budget. Out of this THE, the LTC sector received less than $1 billion USD, further emphasizing the limited financial support that the LTC sector receives. By the end of 2020, healthcare funding is estimated to reach $16.1 billion USD, which is an 8.7% increase. However, there are still no clear statistics in the healthcare sector regarding the financial allocation committed to LTC needs in the same period. In the wake of COVID-19, one can anticipate that the demand for LTC services will rise, illustrating the need to prioritize LTC financing and resource allocation.

In the future, projected financial spending is forecast to rise to $18.3 billion USD by 2023, which is about 6% annual growth in healthcare funding. A 10-year forecast to 2030 projects that healthcare expenditure will rise to $29 billion USD. Mean healthcare spending is expected to account for 3.7% of the UAE's GDP by 2030, which is a gradual increase from 3.4% based on estimations by the Business Monitor International (BMI) group (Export.gov., 2020; Hussein & Ismail, 2018; Unroe et al., 2017). The new health insurance program has supported efforts to advance UAE healthcare under Daman. In Dubai, government-funded payer schemes have benefited up to 130,000 individuals by offering access to 23 private hospitals and more than 500 medical clinics in Dubai. In 2016, the DHA directed all Dubai residents to ensure they had health insurance coverage, a directive that was tied to the renewal and issuance of their UAE residence visas (Export.gov., 2020).

3.2. Health Services Financing

Health functions are the services delivered by providers and include curative (inpatient, home or daycare, and outpatient) and rehabilitative services, LTC, ancillary services, medical goods, prevention, and public health services, and health administration and governance services. Curative services, ancillary services, medical goods, and preventive services accounted for 55%, 14%, 20%, and 6% of CHE in 2012, respectively.

3.2.1. Curative Services

Data on financial spending on health functions in the UAE show that curative services account for the most spending on health, at about 55% of CHE. Inpatient, home care, and outpatient services accounted for 30%, 12%, and 23% of CHE in 2019, respectively (Burchardt, Jones, & Obolenskaya, 2018; Jaffe, 2019; Zeng et al., 2020). The major contributor to spending on curative services is the local government (40%), followed by voluntary insurance (35%) and households (22%), while the federal government pays 3%. About 64% of CHE spent on curative services was spent by hospitals (78% of inpatient care, 83% of curative homecare, and 45% of outpatient curative services), and 20% by providers of ambulatory health care (5% of curative daycare and 47% of curative outpatient care) (UAE Government, 2020).

3.2.2. Rehabilitation Services

With less relevance in the functional structure is rehabilitative care, which had a share of just 1% of CHE. The major contributor to spending on rehabilitation services was the local government (69%), followed by voluntary insurance (20%), with 12% paid by households. About 75% of CHE spent on rehabilitation services were spent in hospitals, and 22% were spent in ambulatory health care facilities (UAE Government, 2020). Spending on rehabilitation services includes both long-term service providers and ancillary services. In terms of LTC funding, the proportion of CHE reported to have been spent on long-term nursing shows a striking range, from less than 1% in Dubai to 4% in Abu Dhabi, to 7% in Sharjah, and 8% in Ajman and Fujairah. The UAE spent 1.02% of CHE (2 million AED) on LTC, compared to 11% for OECD countries. Some of the variation in spending on LTC among different Emiratis may be attributed to overestimation or underestimation in some procedures (Kümpel & Schneider, 2020). For example, the high share in Abu Dhabi reflects an overestimation, since it includes expenditure on accommodation in all nursing and residential facilities for older people, not only in nursing homes; the low share in Dubai is partly due to the greater role of informal care by private home care providers and the lack of data sources concerning the service codes provided in the LTC social care sector (UAE Government, 2020).

3.2.3. Ancillary Services

In terms of ancillary services financing, available data reveals that funding accounted for 14% of the CHE. The major contributor to spending on ancillary services is voluntary insurance (56%), followed by households (21%), then local governments (20%), and the federal government (3%) (Garrow, 2020). About 35% of CHE spent on ancillary services were spent in hospitals (35% to laboratory services and 47% to imaging services), 24% was spent by providers of ambulatory health care (30% was spent on laboratory services and 19% was spent on imaging services), and 26% was spent by providers of ancillary services (17% was spent on laboratory services and 18% was spent on imaging services) (Del Pozo-Rubio & Jiménez-Rubio, 2019; Foster et al., 2019; Graham & Bilger, 2017).

3.2.4. Medical Products and Pharmaceuticals

The financing of medical products consumed 20% of the CHE in 2018. Households contribute about 29% of expenditures on medical goods (588 million AED), of which about 86% (508 million AED) is spent in the retail sector. Household spending on medical goods (508 million AED) constitutes about 68% of the total amount of money spent in the retail sector (745 million AED), indicating both relatively high volumes of consumption and high cost. Patients pay very high prices for medicines when purchased from private retail pharmacies in the UAE, and the cost of original brands were found to be 23.5 times higher than the international reference price (WHO, 2010). Nevertheless, generics still account for only 15% of the pharmaceutical market, which is a significantly lower percentage than in many other countries. The recorded spending pattern in the UAE is likely due to self-prescribing practices and over-prescription of pharmaceuticals by providers, which may indicate that patients demand medication that is not clinically indicated and ask private pharmacies to prescribe it (Hamidi, 2015).

Globally, 20%–40% of human and financial resources spent on health are wasted. Common causes of inefficiency include demotivated health workers, duplication of services, and inappropriate use or overuse of medicines and technologies. By far, this indicates the need to control health spending in the pharmaceutical sector and to monitor the use of medicines in retail pharmacies (Lorenz-Dant, 2020). In the past six years, the UAE federal government has taken steps to reduce the relatively high prices of patented drugs and to boost generic markets, with some success (UAE Government, 2020). The MOH managed to reduce the prices of medicines after talks aiming to unify branded medicine prices across the GCC states. Currently, prices of patented medicines are more in line with those of comparator countries than they used to be.

3.3. LTC Financing in the UAE

LTC financing for older people in the UAE is largely supported by the government through annual budgetary allocation to healthcare. In both Dubai and Abu Dhabi, around 70% of outpatient LTC visits are made to private healthcare facilities, while for inpatient activity in private clinics the proportion is about 60% in Dubai and 40% in Abu Dhabi (Del Pozo-Rubio & Jiménez-Rubio, 2019). In the other five Emiratis, the MOH acts as both the regulator and as the main provider of LTC care services. Available data from 2018 shows that there are 41 government facilities and 83 private hospitals in the UAE that provide LTC services, representing an increase of 25% since 2010 (Del Pozo-Rubio & Jiménez-Rubio, 2019). A recent WHO report on chronic care and LTC service provision shows that in the last decade, the UAE has recorded a 16% increase in LTC financing, with the sector largely focusing on home care and nursing homes (Pozo-Rubio, Pardo-García, & Escribano-Sotos, 2020; WHO, 2015).

In Abu Dhabi, LTC financing has been boosted by mandatory health insurance for all expatriates and nationals based on the 2015 healthcare reforms of national insurance coverage (Shaikh et al., 2016). There are three broad categories of health insurance in the UAE: Thiqa, basic, and enhanced. The Thiqa plan, in which all Abu Dhabi nationals have been required to enroll since 2008, provides comprehensive coverage at no cost to plan participants. The remaining two plans are directed towards expatriates residing in the emirate. As the first emirate to introduce a compulsory medical insurance scheme for expatriate workers in 2006, Abu Dhabi has long been a leader in the health care sector. Since then, the UAE has continued to implement changes to improve the LTC insurance system, including a 2010 decision to require all hospitals and insurers to bill LTC-based services on diagnosis-related groups (DRGs) by the end of 2011. The expectation is that over time, such LTC billing will improve efficiency in the provision of LTC in the UAE.

The basic plan is the mandatory minimum LTC coverage, offered at the government-subsidized price of Dh600 AED per year (Abduelkarem et al., 2020). Alternatively, non-nationals also have the option of enrolling in an enhanced plan, which provides additional coverage, but premiums are set by the market (Malik et al., 2020). The Thiqa and basic plans are administered by Daman, a government-owned, specialized health insurance company that was set up in 2005, while enhanced plans are offered by a variety of private sector players in addition to Daman (Moonesar et al., 2018). In line with LTC service provision, the three health insurance models in the UAE also determine how providers, such as physicians, hospitals and labs, are reimbursed for every LTC service delivered. For LTC expatriate patients that are covered by the basic plan, the government sets the tariffs that providers receive.

For LTC services rendered to expatiates enrolled in one of the enhanced plans, private sector insurance companies and providers negotiate payments for each of the LTC services. For Thiqa plan participants, the health care provider for various services is paid the equivalent of the highest rate negotiated under Daman's enhanced plans. However, any additional charges are covered by individuals through out-of-pocket payments. In 2018, there were over 15.3 million insurance claims, out of which 25% are claims based on LTC and clinic services, with the cost of each claim being $105 for a total LTC insurance bill of $1.6 billion USD. As of 2019, the LTC claims have grown to over 2 million but with a reduced total bill of $1.5 billion USD annually, according to a recent report by the Health Authority Abu Dhabi (2019). Therefore, the approximate annual LTC spending in the UAE is $1.5 billion, representing a decline from $105 in 2017 to about $98 per individual reimbursement in 2019 (Abduelkarem et al., 2020).

Despite the steady rise in the number of LTC claims and the overall cost, some scholars have noted that the decrease per individual appropriate, considering that standardized regulation and payment rules, transport, and universal health insurance coverage allow for better control of costs. Besides, proper financing ensures that LTC health needs are met and that UAE patients have the freedom to choose their LTC provider (Pozo-Rubio, Pardo-García, & Escribano-Sotos, 2020). By contrast, other researchers have cautioned that increasing LTC costs and claims signal the need for additional changes to LTC financing to ensure its sustainability (Arsenijevic et al., 2016; Health Authority Abu Dhabi, 2019; Zeng et al., 2020).

According to the WHO (2020), estimations for the UAE reveal that the government spent 25% of its total healthcare budget on covering medical costs for overseas treatment, where one thirds of the cases were related to LTC services (Abu-Saad, Bejjani, & Fares, 2019; Khan, Hussein, & Deane, 2017). Thus, there are growing concerns that the high percentage of patients travelling overseas for LTC care implies possible shortcomings in UAE service quality and resource allocation for LTC care. For instance, the DHA sponsored 2,717 patients in 2018 for medical treatment abroad, which is an increase of 583 in 3 years (Dubai Health Authority, 2016). In 2019, the HAAD sponsored 1,932 patients for different overseas treatments (Dubai Health Authority, 2019; Hussein & Ismail, 2018). The rising number of overseas treatments raises concerns about the effectiveness of the current LTC services in meeting demands of its citizens. Thus, additional resource allocation and financial investment is needed to reduce the cost of overseas treatment by developing local capacity in handling and managing LTC services.

4. Addressing Future LTC Financing Challenge

Having an adequate system of LTC financing in the UAE is a pre-condition for translating the need for care and services into effective demand. An effective design of a financing model for the UAE should have three main elements: (1) the source of finance; (2) the rules defining eligible target groups and forms of care services provided; and (3) the system of payment for service provision, which is linked with the delivery system. Spending levels for LTC services need to be streamlined where medical and social care should be combined. However, the expenditures for LTC remain relatively small (at $98 per claim annually) compared to general health services and public pension systems, that are $2500-$6,372 per patient on annual basis. These insights show that currently, the UAE prioritizes healthcare financing where the annual coverage is relatively high, averaging $4,436, compared to the LTC average of $101.5 between 2017 and 2019.

The limited budgetary allocation to LTC implies that the UAE is unable to adequately meet the LTC of most patients, a challenge that may help explain why one third of the overseas medical costs are attributed to chronic care and long-term needs (Abu-Saad, Bejjani, & Fares, 2019; Khan, Hussein, & Deane, 2017; WHO, 2020). In addition, the low number of hospital beds dedicated to LTC services further complicates any potential commitment towards improving the current LTC care needs of nationals. When compounded with the LTC needs of expatriates, it becomes clear that the existing resource allocation and service delivery is insufficient. There is a need for additional financial support, resource allocation such as beds, and hiring of medical personnel to meet the growing LTC needs in the UAE. Besides, lack of specific regulation of LTC services means the UAE MOH should to create a specific healthcare department dedicated towards meeting LTC needs. Table 1 presents important strategies that the UAE may take into consideration when designing a sustainable LTC financing model.

Experience from OECD countries demonstrates that, historically, the amount of public financing for LTC largely depends on how much a society can rely on informal care. Factors having a long-term impact on the need for care for older people and expenditure levels are the ratio of older people to the working-age population, disease prevention and health promotion, household structure, female labor force participation, and migration patterns.

Table 1. Alternative elements to consider when designing a sustainable LTC financing model in the UAE

Factors to Consider	Assessments
Source of finance	• Tax-based (Nordic European countries) • Public, compulsory LTC social insurance models (Germany, the Netherlands, Luxembourg, Japan, and the Republic of Korea) • Co-payment by clients (a common requirement in many countries which may vary by care setting)
Eligible target group	• Universal coverage • Means-tested, based on strict income or asset tests to set financial thresholds for eligibility for publicly funded care • Level of need according to needs assessment
Forms of services	• Homecare • Community care (daycare centers) • Institutional (residential) care
Payment for service provision	• To eligible clients: cash payment or in-kind services, vouchers • To service providers: payment for time, services, or outcomes

Source: Author.

In the UAE, the role of the government as the primary LTC financier has materialized in the high-level funding allocated to the older populations and persons with chronic needs. To further stimulate private sector development of services for LTC financing, the government remains committed to allocating LTC resources. Most of these measures are intended to address the financing of LTC for individual consumers. Table 2 summarizes common LTC funding approaches that might be considered in the UAE, based on their advantages and disadvantages.

Considering future LTC financing in the UAE, a key aspect to contemplate is that public finance is a pre-condition for building a service market with wide coverage that is accessible for all clients in need and where consumers can exercise their choices. In OECD countries, LTC is based on stable public financial resources (either tax-based or social insurance-based). Financial pressure has led to gradual adjustments, but the basics of the wide coverage of quality services have been maintained. To increase the coverage and quality of LTC services in the UAE, an effective and sustainable public financing system needs to be established to reduce overreliance on natural resources. A mix of public and private payments should be designed and implemented. An important issue in the development of a robust public financing system in the UAE would be the division of responsibilities for financing among the different layers of government.

Table 2. Advantages and Disadvantages of Financing Approaches to LTC Care

Approach	**Advantages**	**Disadvantages**
Mandatory social insurance (Germany, Korea, Rep., Japan)	Entitlement to benefit affordable contribution (if income-related)	Limited tax base Rigidity in benefits awarded Implicit debt
Tax-based, universal systems	Broader tax base	No direct link between revenues and benefits Less transparency in benefit allocation Implicit debt
Private insurance	Theoretically neutral for the public budget	If voluntary: • Not affordable for people with low, insecure income • Adverse selection (If mandatory, may require subsidies for people with low incomes)

Source: Author.

In the short run, a tax-based system with eligibility based on need (defined as a combination of the severity of limited functional ability and resources) may be an appropriate LTC financing framework for the UAE, but a social insurance-based system would be most appropriate in the long term, considering risks of potential pandemics such as COVID-19. A logical next step would be for the government to widen the safety net to cover a greater number of older people most in need of LTC and direct public resources to them. The support needs to be targeted at specific groups such as homeless, jobless, very old, frail, and isolated persons without consistent application of a need's assessment. While the funds are barely enough to cover significant amounts of LTC in the UAE, they do improve the financial position of people who are at a high risk of needing LTC. In terms of spending on LTC relative to GDP, public spending is expected to increase to improve the depth and quality of care coverage in the UAE.

Conclusion

The findings of this study point to potential opportunities for growth and improvement in several health policy issues, including increasing focus and funding of LTC services, shifting from inpatient care to outpatient and home-based services, and strengthening LTC financing options while introducing cost-containment measures. Despite the continued annual increase in healthcare financing, there is a decline of financial and resource allocation for LTC services, making it difficult to deliver the much-needed care to patients. Besides, the lack of an LTC-specific department in the UAE healthcare sector means that urgent LTC needs are not prioritized, resulting in a large number of LTC patients travelling overseas to seek better care services. Dedicating a department within the healthcare sector would help prioritize LTC needs in terms of regulating the sector; committing the needed financial resources through the annual budget; and ensuring appropriate financial allocation, resource allocation, and the hiring of personnel who are dedicated to LTC delivery and independent from primary and secondary healthcare systems. Spending on inpatient services remains the highest-costing component of CHE in the UAE. More care is often not better care, and inpatient care is highly labor-intensive and expensive. Reorientation of the health system is needed to reduce the share of spending on inpatient services for LTC patients and move in favor of day surgery, outpatient, and home-based services. Reforming LTC payment mechanisms will influence the incentives and behaviors of both patients and providers within the UAE, where more patients could seek local services as opposed to travelling overseas for medical treatment. LTC financing reforms through the introduction of the LTC regulatory and financing framework that is independent from the current healthcare model (Thiqa, basic and enhanced) holds the potential to improve LTC service provision and delivery in the UAE for both Emirati nationals and expatriates.

REFERENCES

Abduelkarem, A., Sharif, S., Bankessli, F., Kamal, S., Kulhasan, N., & Hamrouni, A. (2020). Obesity and its associated risk factors among school-aged children in Sharjah, UAE. *PLoS ONE*, 15(6), e0234244. https://doi.org/10.1371/journal.pone.0234244.

Abu-Saad Huijer, H., Bejjani, R., & Fares, S. (2019). Quality of care, spirituality, relationships, and finances in older adult palliative care patients in Lebanon. *Annals of Palliative Medicine*, 8(5), 551-558. doi: http://dx.doi.org/10.21037/apm.2019.09.08.

Alao, D., Cevik, A., Eid, H., Jummani, Z., & Abu-Zidan, F. (2020). Trauma system developments reduce mortality in hospitalized trauma patients in Al-Ain City, United Arab Emirates, despite increased severity of injury. *World Journal of Emergency Surgery*, 15(1). doi: 10.1186/s13017-020-00327-y.

Albarrán, I., Alonso-González, P., & Grané, A. (2019). Long term care insurance pricing in Spanish population: a functional data approach. *The European Journal of Finance*, 26(2-3), 258-276. doi: 10.1080/ 1351847x.2019.1678497.

AlKetbi, L. M. B., Grivna, M., & Al Dhaheri, S. (2020). Risky driving behaviour in Abu Dhabi, United Arab Emirates: a cross-sectional, survey-based study. *BMC Public Health*, 20(1). doi:10.1186/s12889-020-09389-8.

AlQutob R, Moonesar IA, Tarawneh MR, Al Nsour M, Khader Y. (2020). Public health strategies for a gradual public sector lockdown lifting in Jordan and United Arab Emirates during COVID-19 crisis. *JMIR Public Health and Surveillance*. 26/06/2020:20478.

Arsenijevic, J., Pavlova, M., Rechel, B., & Groot, W. (2016). Catastrophic health care expenditure among older people with chronic diseases in

15 European countries. *PLoS ONE*, 11(7) doi: http://dx.doi.org/10.1371/journal.pone.0157765.

Barczyk, D., & Kredler, M. (2019). Long-Term Care Across Europe and the United States: The Role of Informal and Formal Care. *Fiscal Studies*, 40(3), 329-373. doi: 10.1111/1475-5890.12200.

Burchardt, T., Jones, E., & Obolenskaya, P. (2018). Formal and informal long-term care in the community: Interlocking or incoherent systems? *Journal of Social Policy*, 47(3), 479-503. doi: http://dx.doi.org/10.1017/S0047279417000903.

Campbell, J. (2014). Japan's Long-Term Care Insurance System. *Eldercare Policies in Japan And Scandinavia*, 9-30. doi: 10.1057/978 1137402639_2.

Del Pozo-Rubio, R., & Jiménez-Rubio, D. (2019). Catastrophic risk associated with out-of-pocket payments for long term care in Spain. *Health Policy*, 123(6), 582-589. doi: http://dx.doi.org/10.1016/j.healthpol.2019.03.016.

Department of Health - Abu Dhabi. (2019). *Healthcare Capacity Master Plan.*

Dubai Statistics Centre. (2016). *Estimated population number by nationality - Emirate of Dubai.* 2016. https://www.dsc.gov.ae/Publication/Population%20Bulletin%20Emirate%20of%20Dubai%202016.pdf.

Dubai Health Authority. (2017). *Dubai Annual Health Statistical Report 2016.*

Export.gov. (2020). *Healthcare Resource Guide: United Arab Emirates.* Retrieved 25 August 2020, from https://2016.export.gov/industry/health/healthcareresourceguide/eg_main_108626.asp.

Fasseeh, A., Karam, R., Jameleddine, M., George, M., Kristensen, F., & Al-Rabayah, A. et al., (2020). Implementation of Health Technology Assessment in the Middle East and North Africa: Comparison Between the Current and Preferred Status. *Frontiers in Pharmacology*, 11. doi: 10.3389/fphar.2020.00015.

Favreault, M. M., Gleckman, H., & Johnson, R. W. (2015). Financing long-term services and supports: Options reflect trade- offs for older

Americans and federal spending. *Health Affairs*, 34(12), 2181-0_1,1-29. doi: http://dx.doi.org/10.1377/hlthaff.2015.1226.

Foster, C. C., Agrawal, R. K., & Davis, M. M. (2019). Home health care for children with medical complexity: Workforce gaps, policy, and future directions. *Health Affairs*, 38(6), 987-993. doi: http://dx.doi.org/10.1377/hlthaff.2018.05531.

Gaili, Aiman & Awlaqi, Ahmed & Hammadeh, Mohamad Eid & Koornneef, Erik. (2019). *The Impact of Co-Payments on Individual Access to Long-term Care Services in the United Arab Emirates in Comparison to the Middle East*.

Garrow, Renee. (2020). *Health Effects of Spousal Caregiving among Elderly Americans. Undergraduate Honours Theses. Paper 1484.* https://scholarworks.wm.edu/honorstheses/1484.

Gachiri, W. (2017). A Gradient Analysis of Economic Development and Chronic Diseases. Case of Diabetes and Life expectancy in United Arab Emirates. *Journal of Applied Business and Economics*, 19 (1); pp. 35-43.

Graham, W. C. K., & Bilger, M. (2017). Financing long-term services and supports: Ideas from Singapore. *The Milbank Quarterly*, 95(2), 358-407. doi: http://dx.doi.org/10.1111/1468-0009.12264.

Jaffe, S. (2019). Home health care providers struggle with state laws and Medicare rules as demand rises. *Health Affairs*, 38(6), 981-986. doi: http://dx.doi.org/10.1377/hlthaff.2019.00529.

Hamidi S. (2015). Health services financing and delivery: analysis of policy options for Dubai, United Arab Emirates. *ClinicoEconomics and Outcomes Research: CEOR*, 7, 133–143. https://doi.org/10.2147/CEOR.S75743.

Health Authority Abu Dhabi. (2019). *Health statistics 2019*. Abu Dhabi: Health Authority Abu Dhabi; [cited 7th July 2020] Available at: http://www.haad.ae/HAAD/LinkClick.aspx?fileticket=KeJK5ZsIuns%3d&tabid=1516.

Harrington, C., Armstrong, H., Halladay, M., Havig, A., Jacobsen, F., & MacDonald, M. et al., (2015). Comparison of Nursing Home Financial

Transparency and Accountability in Four Locations. *Ageing International*, 41(1), 17-39. doi: 10.1007/s12126-015-9233-3.

Health Authority Abu Dhabi. (2018). *Health statistics 2017.* Abu Dhabi: Department of Health.

Health Authority Abu Dhabi (2017). *Capacity Master Plan.* Abu Dhabi; 2016. www.haad.ae/statistics.

Heger, D., & Korfhage, T. (2018). Care choices in Europe: To each according to his or her needs?: The journal of health care organization, provision, and financing the journal of health care organization, provision, and financing. *Inquiry*, 55 doi: http://dx.doi.org/10.1177/0046958018780848.

Hussein, S., & Ismail, M. (2018). Ageing and elderly care in the Arab region: Policy challenges and opportunities. *Ageing International*, 42(3), 274-289. doi: http://dx.doi.org/10.1007/s12126-016-9244-8.

Khan, H., Hussein, S., & Deane, J. (2018). Nexus between Demographic Change and Elderly Care Need in the Gulf Cooperation Council (GCC) Countries: Some Policy Implications. *Ageing International*, 42(4), 466-487. doi: 10.1007/s12126-017-9303-9.

Koornneef EJ, Robben PBM, Al Seiari MB, et al., (2012). Health system reform in the emirate of Abu Dhabi. *Health Policy*. 2012;108(2–3):115–21. 10.1016/j. healthpol.2012.08.026.

Koornneef, E., Robben, P., & Blair, I. (2017). Progress and outcomes of health systems reform in the United Arab Emirates: a systematic review. *BMC Health Services Research*, 17(1). doi: 10.1186/s12913-017-2597-1.

Kümpel, C., & Schneider, U. (2020). Additional reimbursement for outpatient physicians treating nursing home residents reduces avoidable hospital admissions: Results of a reimbursement change in Germany. *Health Policy*, 124(4), 470-477. doi: 10.1016/j.healthpol.2020.02.009.

Lapão LV. (2018). The Future Impact of Healthcare Services Digitalization on Health Workforce: The Increasing Role of Medical Informatics. *Stud Health Technol Inform.*, 228:675-679.

Lehnert, T., Heuchert, M., Hussain, K., & König, H. (2019). Stated preferences for long-term care: A literature review. *Ageing and Society*, 39(9), 1873-1913. doi: http://dx.doi.org/10.1017/S014468 6X18000314.

Lindström, C., Rosvall, M., & Lindström, M. (2019). Unmet healthcare needs and mortality: A prospective cohort study from southern Sweden. *Scandinavian Journal of Public Health*, 48(3), 267-274. doi: 10.1177/1403494819863530.

Lorenz-Dant, K. (2020) Germany and the COVID-19 long-term care situation. LTC covid, *International Long-Term Care Policy Network*, CPEC-LSE, 26 May 2020.

Lord, J., Davlyatov, G., Thomas, K. S., Hyer, K., & Weech-Maldonado, R. (2018). The role of assisted living capacity on nursing home financial performance: The journal of health care organization, provision, and financing the journal of health care organization, provision, and financing. *Inquiry*, 55 doi: http://dx.doi.org/10.1177/0046958018 793285.

Malik, D., Malik, Y., Chander, R., Singh, J., Singh, T., & Bansal, K. et al., (2020). Association between Knowledge and Drug Adherence among Patients with Hypertension in Abu Dhabi, Sharjah and Ajman-UAE. *Current Topics In Medicine And Medical Research* Vol. 2, 3(2), 67-89. https://doi.org/10.9734/bpi/ctmamr/v2.

Meinow, B., Wastesson, J., Kåreholt, I., & Kelfve, S. (2020). Long-Term Care Use During the Last 2 Years of Life in Sweden: Implications for Policy to Address Increased Population Aging. *Journal Of The American Medical Directors Association*, 21(6), 799-805. doi: 10.1016/j.jamda.2020.01.003.

Moonesar, I. A., Elshokamy, M. M., & Sayani, H. (2018). The State of UAE Healthcare Service Delivery: Public Perceptions Preliminary Insights. *UAE Public Policy*. pp. 1-112.

Nadash, P., Doty, P., & von Schwanenflügel, M. (2017). The German Long-Term Care Insurance Program: Evolution and Recent Developments. *The Gerontologist*, 58(3), 588-597. doi: 10.1093/ geront/gnx018.

Orlovic, M., Marti, J., & Mossialos, E. (2017). Analysis of end-of-life care, out-of-pocket spending, and place of death in 16 European countries and Israel. *Health Affairs*, 36(7), 1201. doi: http://dx.doi.org/10.1377/hlthaff.2017.0166.

Paulo, M. S., Loney, T., & Lapão, L. V. (2019). How do we strengthen the health workforce in a rapidly developing high-income country? A case study of Abu Dhabi's health system in the United Arab Emirates. *Human resources for health*, 17(1), 9. https://doi.org/10.1186/s12960-019-0345-9.

Paulo, M. R. (2019). *The chronic care model use in the emirate of Abu Dhabi health system: is it enough to address the growing problem of chronic diseases?* Instituto de Higiene e Medicina Tropical.

Pearson, C. F., Quinn, C. C., Loganathan, S., Datta, A. R., Mace, B. B., & Grabowski, D. C. (2019). The forgotten middle: Many middle-income seniors will have insufficient resources for housing and health care. *Health Affairs*, 38(5), 851-12. doi: http://dx.doi.org/10.1377/hlthaff.2018.05233.

Pozo-Rubio, R., Pardo-García, I., & Escribano-Sotos, F. (2020). Financial catastrophism inherent with out-of-pocket payments in long term care for households: A latent impoverishment. International *Journal of Environmental Research and Public Health*, 17(1) doi: http://dx.doi.org/10.3390/ijerph17010295.

Shaikh AS, Irshad B, Yyagi H et al., (2016). *Investment big bets health care and life sciences in the GCC*. London: Ernst & Young Global Limited; [cited 7th July 2020] Available at: http://www.ey.com/Publication/vwLUAssets/EYinvestment-big-bets-healthcare-tl-report/$FILE/EY-investment-big-betshealthcare-tl-report.pdf.

Tuite, A., Bogoch, I., Sherbo, R., Watts, A., Fisman, D., & Khan, K. (2020). Estimation of Coronavirus Disease 2019 (COVID-19) Burden and Potential for International Dissemination of Infection from Iran. *Annals of Internal Medicine*, 172(10), 699-701. doi: 10.7326/m20-0696.

UAE Government. (2020). *Healthcare budget - The Official Portal of the UAE Government*. Retrieved 25 August 2020, from https://u.ae/en/information-and-services/health-and-fitness/healthcare-budget.

Unroe, K. T., Bernard, B., Stump, T. E., Tu, W., & Callahan, C. M. (2017). Variation in hospice services by location of care: Nursing home versus assisted living facility versus home. *Journal of the American Geriatrics Society*, 65(7), 1490-1496. doi: 10.1111/jgs.14826.

Vetter P, Boecker K. (2012). Benefits of a single payment system: case study of Abu Dhabi health system reforms. *Health Policy*. 2012;108(2–3), 105-114. 10.1016/j. healthpol.2012.08.009.

World Health Organization. (2015). *World Health Statistics 2015*. Geneva: World Health Organization; 2015 [cited 2016 Aug 11] Available at: http://apps.who.int/iris/bitstream/10665/170250/1/9789240694439_eng.pdf.

World Health Organization. (2020). *Health workforce snapshot United Arab Emirates*. https://apps.who.int/iris/bitstream/handle/10665/332425/WHOEMHRH648E-.

World Health Organization. (2019) *Framework for action for health workforce development*. 2019. http://www.emro.who.int/images/stories/hrh/Strategic_framework_for_health_workforce_development_MAY_2019_3.pdf.

Yeh, M. (2019). Long-term care system in Taiwan: the 2017 major reform and its challenges. *Ageing and Society*, 40(6), 1334-1351. doi: 10.1017/s0144686x18001745.

Zeng, Q., Wang, Q., Zhang, L., & Xu, X. (2020). Comparison of the measurement of long-term care costs between china and other countries: A systematic review of the last decade. *Healthcare*, 8(2), 117. doi: http://dx.doi.org/10.3390/healthcare8020117.

In: The Future of Long-Term Care
Editor: Pablo Villalobos Dintrans
ISBN: 978-1-53619-263-6

Chapter 6

TOWARDS A LONG-TERM CARE SYSTEM IN MEXICO

Emmanuel González-Bautista[1,*], Luis Miguel F. Gutiérrez-Robledo[2], Mariana López-Ortega[2,†] and Eduardo Sosa-Tinoco[2]
[1]Gerontopole of Toulouse, Institute of Aging,
Toulouse University Hospital (CHU Toulouse),
Toulouse, France
[2]National Institute of Geriatrics (INGER),
National Institutes of Health,
Mexico City, Mexico

ABSTRACT

It is expected that disability and care dependence will increase in Mexico as a result of the accelerated demographic aging process coupled with high prevalence of chronic non-communicable diseases, frailty, and adverse socioeconomic conditions.

* Corresponding Author's E-mail: emmanuel.gonzalez-bautista@univ-tlse3.fr.
† Corresponding Author's E-mail: marianalopezortega@gmail.com.

In a context of institutional fragmentation, lack of a regulatory framework regarding outside-of-hospital care, and a majority of long-term care (LTC) provided by families in Mexico (non-paid care activities reached 23.5% of the GDP in 2018), it is urgent to foster the discussion with stakeholders to advance on the design and later implementation of an LTC system with a community-based approach.

Data from the Mexican Health and Aging Study (MHAS) show that 22% of people 60 years and older reported experiencing difficulties in performing at least one of the activities of daily living (ADLs) and almost 15% at least one of the instrumental activities of daily living (IADLs). In those aged 80 and over, there was a 44% prevalence of ADLs disability, with women having higher prevalence of difficulties than men.

Growing demand for LTC services coexists with the absence of a national regulatory entity to oversee management and quality of care standards for LTC services and to monitor and evaluate LTC providers. In section 1 of our chapter, we present an overview of the current institutional architecture of LTC providers in Mexico, despite the lack of precise information on the total number of public or private permanent and temporary care institutions available in the country.

In section 2, we define the LTC system as the connected set of all the resources efficiently shared between the health and social sectors to satisfy the demand for services linked to care as a human right. We propose three major connecting nodes that will be at the core of the linkage between the health, social, and other involved sectors in the design of an LTC care system in Mexico: 1) human capital, 2) material capital (financing/infrastructure), and 3) meta-capital (data and information).

Section 3 presents some of the lessons learned during the COVID-19 epidemic in Mexico regarding the necessary preparedness for the LTC systems in the face of future pandemics.

Finally, in section 4 we summarize some multisectoral and health-specific pending tasks to advance on the design and implementation of an LTC system in Mexico in terms of research, care provision, and regulatory framework.

1. The Context of Long-term Care in Mexico

Mexico is ageing rapidly, and its older population is expected to nearly triple, from 6.3% of the total population in the year 2010 to almost 22.6% by 2050. For the first time in 2015, the number of people aged 60 years and older was larger than those aged 0 to 4 years old (Instituto Nacional de

Estadística y Geografía, 2015). This transition was brought by a sharp decline in global fertility rates and mortality, an increase in public health interventions, and better access to health care services, resulting in important gains in life expectancy. In the year 2018, life expectancy in Mexico was 75 years, 72 for men and 78 for women (United Nations Population Division, n.d.).

However, this ageing process is taking place in a context of wide economic disparities, few public economic support programs for older people, and a constant reliance on unpaid family support to provide economic security and health and personal care for older people (Gutiérrez-Robledo, López-Ortega, & Arango-Lopera, 2012).

In addition, Mexico is experiencing a rapidly changing social context characterized by the transformation of the roles of women, smaller families, and increasing participation of women in the workforce. This has reduced the total number of potential caregivers and the time that they have available to provide unpaid care for older people and people with temporary or permanent disabilities (Huenchuan-Navarro & Rodríguez-Velázquez, 2015). On the other hand, societal reliance on unpaid family care, given the limited availability of formal long-term care (LTC) services, continues to affect women's labor force participation, with negative effects on the economy and increased gender inequality (Cafagna et al., 2019).

It is clear that the need to generate optimal health care services and public care policies for older people, including LTC, is now more relevant than ever. Care is a fundamental part of the fabric of any society, and therefore constitutes a central element in the social development and wellbeing of older people and those with care dependency (Huenchuan-Navarro & Rodríguez-Velázquez, 2015; López-Ortega & Aranco, 2019).

1.1. Long-Term Care Needs

Care needs or dependency has been defined in many ways in recent years, to identify the best ways to provide services or focus programs. For example, in a recent study on care policy in Mexico City, Huenchuan Navarro & Rodríguez Velázquez (2015) describe the care scenario for older people with respect to other groups needing care (such as infants and young children), in terms of their age, their functional disability, or the help they need to perform daily and instrumental activities of daily living (IADLs).

While the majority of older people are functional and independent and age is not the sole factor causing functional disability and care dependency, studies in different countries have documented how difficulty to perform daily activities increases with age, especially for those in their eighties. For Mexico, studies have shown that it is after 75 years of age that the presence of disability and frailty have a clear relationship with chronological age (Díaz-Venegas, De La Vega, & Wong, 2015; García-Peña, Ávila-Funes, Dent, Gutiérrez-Robledo, & Pérez-Zepeda, 2016; López-Ortega & Aranco, 2019; López-Ortega & Jiménez-Bolón, 2015).

However, given the negative impact of chronic diseases, especially if untreated or not correctly managed, the definition of care dependency based on difficulty performing activities of daily living (ADLs) or IADLs in addition to age has been defined as a more accurate input in generating care policies. Data from the Mexican Health and Aging Study (MHAS) show that 22% of people 60 years and older reported experiencing difficulties in performing at least one of the ADLs, and almost 15% at least one of the IADLs, with women having a higher prevalence of difficulties than men. Difficulties also increase with age: while 15% of those in the 60-69 years group have difficulties performing ADLs, this prevalence reaches 44% in the 80 years and older group. These patterns are also seen in performing IADLs. Finally, as age increases, people report higher prevalence of difficulty performing more than one activity, and there is a difference in the prevalence of difficulty depending on the specific activity; making purchases, walking, and getting in and out of bed had the highest prevalence of difficulty (López-Ortega & Aranco, 2019).

In terms of planning and development of care policies, it is important to take all these characteristics into account, as they define different needs that must respond to different support strategies.

1.2. Supply of Long-Term Care for Older people in Mexico

Mexico does not have a publicly financed LTC system, nor does it have a national-level mandatory registry of institutions, e.g., an information system to count, monitoring, and regulate them. In addition, there is a complete absence of a national regulatory body to oversee management and quality of care standards for LTC services as well as monitoring, accreditation, and evaluation of LTC providers. This has generated an absence of precise information on the total number of public or private permanent and temporary care institutions available in the country, and there is little documentation of the characteristics and conditions of care homes, including the impact on residents' wellbeing.

There are some permanent LTC residences (care homes) for older people in the country. An ongoing analysis at the National Institute of Geriatrics using the National Economic Units Directory (INEGI, 2014) shows that there are 1,609 facilities. However, there is uncertainty about the type of services they offer, their cost, care quality, and their impact on the well-being and quality of life of residents.

1.2.1. Public LTC Services

With respect to national, publicly funded LTC services, two federal government institutions have a total of ten institutions that provide institutionalized care for older people: the National Institute for Older people (INAPAM) and the National System for the Development of the Family (DIF). INAPAM has six permanent residential institutions (four in the Federal District, one in Guanajuato, and another in Oaxaca) and DIF has four (two in Mexico City, one in the state of Morelos, and one in the state of Oaxaca) (DIF-Transparencia DIF Nacional, 2020; Instituto Nacional de las Personas Adultas Mayores, 2020a). Priority for admission to these public institutions is given to people in extreme conditions of vulnerability, such as older people in situations of abandonment, with no family or close relatives, and without housing. The services are offered at no cost to the resident, generally providing accommodation, food, laundry services, cleaning, general medical care and referral to secondary or tertiary care health services, support with the basic activities of daily life, as well as recreational, sports, and cultural activities. Places that become available in these institutions are offered through a waiting list.

In addition, some municipalities (local public financing) have day centers for older people (mostly recreational). However, given the lack of a national level regulation agency and of a national mandatory registry of institutions, no precise information on the total number of public institutions is available.

1.2.2. Private Long-Term Care Services

Trends shown in local forums suggest that the private LTC sector is growing in the country (INDESOL, presentation 2020). However, the absence of an accreditation and evaluation body means that there is very little standardized information about the type of services provided, their quality, the type of health and care professionals working for them, and their overall impact on the health and wellbeing of the people that live there. The total number of people that use these private services and the size of the private sector are unknown, but one can infer that it is much larger than the public sector, given that the latter only comprises ten residential care institutions for the whole country.

The National Institute of Statistics and Geography (INEGI) and DIF conducted the first Census of Social Assistance Housings (CAAS) in 2015 (INEGI, 2015). Of the 4,517 permanent housing LTC settings included in the CAAS, 1,020 (22.6%) were care homes for older people and a total of 22,611 older persons (identified as resident users) were living in these institutions at the time (INEGI, 2015). Regarding their legal nature, 75% were reported as private non-profit facilities, 8% public (government funded), 2.3% religious associations, and 2% private for-profit institutions. Most non-profit institutions combine multiple financing sources: user fees (78%), personal donations (56%), private sector donations (32%), donations from faith-based organizations (28%), government funds (38%) and selling products made by the residents (3%).

1.2.3. Private Non-Profit Institutions

Most non-profit institutions work under mixed schemes, in which they offer free accommodation services for those older people who do not have resources, nor a family network that supports them, and for those who have limited economic capacity. The group consisting of people without resources generally represents the majority of their residents. For those with economic capacity, recovery fees depending on the available resources of the older person and/or their relatives being charged. To our knowledge, fees in most institutions are established according to the financial situation of the resident through a socio-economic assessment of the older person and their responsible family members, if there are any.

1.2.4. Private for-Profit Institutions

There are also private for-profit institutions that offer care to older people, and while some people become older and increasingly disabled during their time in the institution, most have strict admission requirements that up front only admit "independent" older people with no severe illnesses or disabilities. Their scale, type of services, and quality are not documented, and they vary in quality and costs. While there are institutions that offer common accommodation services in very small spaces, others offer spacious single rooms with an integrated bathroom. Similarly, non-professional caregivers and auxiliary nursing personnel constitute most of the personnel, with very few licensed nurses being hired. For more specialized and personalized nursing care, some institutions allow the resident or family member to hire external personnel for their care when needed, incurring an additional cost. In addition, nursing or other specialized care services contracted out (and paid) by family members are sometimes also allowed. In our experience, some institutions offer a wide range of additional recreational services and amenities, such as cable television, internet, movies, access to a gym, climate and controlled ventilation, or beauty salons.

According to the National Statistics Directory of Economic Units (DENUE), there are 603 private institutions identified as care homes and private homes for the care of the older people. However, there is no additional information to identify if these are for profit or non-profit organizations and as a result, the precise number of private institutions in the country is unknown. Great diversity was found in the total number of private institutions registered in each state of the country (INEGI, 2014).

1.2.5. Private Community Day Care Centers

Just as with permanent LTC settings, there is an increasing market of private day centers. Services provided in day centers are usually focused on independent and highly functional individuals. These are mostly social and recreational centers that aim to maintain the independence and participation of older people, mainly providing occupational therapies, crafts, health promotion and information, training in information and communication technologies (ICTs), physical activity and, in some occasions, general medical and dentist consultations. That is, they focus primarily on functional people and, for the most part, do not consider dependency care as a care strategy or model (López-Ortega & Aranco, 2019). In addition, very few centers focus on groups with specific care needs. For example, with the exception of around 15 day centers for people with dementia in the country, no other day care services are in place for older people (or any other age groups) with disabilities or care dependency.

1.2.6. Other Private Community-Based Services

Recently, technology assisted services and incipient services by care aides at home have been in place, such as at-home personal assistance (not qualified medical care) services provided by private for-profit companies. However, as no regulatory framework or agency exists to establish care standards, monitor, or evaluate these services, little is known on their number and how they operate. Services usually range from basic personal companion services (inside and outside the home) to support with activities of daily living, such as feeding (but not cooking), bathing, basic nursing activities, and physical therapy or rehabilitation. While these services are being offered in Mexico's largest cities, the costs are very high and only accessible to a very small percentage of those who could benefit from them (López-Ortega & Aranco, 2019).

On the other hand, the lack of regulation and standards to overlook these services generates a wide variety with respect to the quality of services provided (including the training and skills of hired personnel), from highly standardized and monitored U.S. franchises operating in Mexico, to agencies/individuals that gather a group of "caregivers" and act as placement services. While the former use highly professional advertising campaigns, services with the latter are usually known from word of mouth. Finally, while it is common practice for domestic workers (day and live-in workers), to provide care on an as-needed basis (for infants, young children, older people, and people with disabilities). No information is publicly available on how many and how much of their time is dedicated to care for each of these population groups.

1.2.7. Unpaid Family Care

Mexico does not have a publicly funded national LTC system, however care is being provided in different ways. Unpaid informal care by family members is the main source of care and in some cases, when economic resources are available, with support from domestic paid workers. As with care to other age groups, unpaid health care for older people is mainly provided by women.

To date, Mexico does not have caregiver surveys or large scale studies that allow for precise estimations on the total number of unpaid family caregivers, their characteristics, nor the type and intensity of care provided. However, as part of Mexico's National Accounts, INEGI estimates on a yearly basis the National Satellite Health Accounts of the Health Sector (Cuenta Satélite del Sector Salud en Mexico, CSSSM), with the aim of estimating the amount of unpaid health and personal care provided (TNRS is its acronym in Spanish) and its value. Data for 2017 (base year 2013) reports that the GDP of the health sector is 5.6% of the national GDP. Of this 5.6%, 1.5% represents unpaid health and personal care performed within the household (INEGI, 2018b). Of this 1.5%, 0.4% corresponds to the value of care for adults 60 years and older (López-Ortega, 2018).

Table 1. General overview of the supply of LTC services in Mexico

	Number of facilities (% where appropriate)	
Latest estimation (national)	1,609	
Public LTC		
INAPAM	6	Permanent housing, mainly for socioeconomically disadvantaged people. Long waiting lists.
DIF	4	
Private LTC		
Country	4,517	permanent housing
For older people	1,020	22.6% (22,611 residents in 2015)
Of which		
Private non-profit		75%
Government funding		8%
Religious associations		2.30%
Private for profit		2%
Non-paid care services		
% of national GDP in 2018		23.5%
% of activities strictly related to health		1.50%
Total time devoted to care related with the basic ADL		
% provided by siblings or grand-children		60%
% provided by the couple		30%
% provided by a hired third party		4%

Source: Authors.

In order to take into account the dimensions of the role of unpaid personal and health work performed within the household, it is important to note that the monetary value of the household's contribution to personal and health care of other household members (27.7%) represents more than half of what is generated by public sector establishments (39.5%), is larger than the contribution of primary care (ambulatory) medical services (17.0%), and is similar to that generated by all hospital services (20.7%) (INEGI, 2018b).

Unpaid household health care for people aged 60 years and over has grown as a proportion of total unpaid household health care in the last seven years (2009-2016), representing 23.5% of the TNRS in 2009 and 25.5% in 2016. The total value of unpaid household health care for people aged 60 years and older in 2016 was 73,679 million pesos (3,905 million USD). As with care for other age groups, home health care for people sixty years of age and over is mainly performed by women, who contributed 72% of the total economic value for an average of 7.2 hours per week, compared to 4.8 hours spent on average by men. Regarding the total time devoted to such care, men performed 32.3%, and women 67.7%. By type of activity, the largest proportion of time was spent on bathing or grooming the older person and feeding or helping him to do so, which represent 43% of the total time dedicated to care (López-Ortega, 2018).

For older people, MHAS data show that of the total care received for basic activities, more than 60% is provided by children, sons/daughters-in-law, or grandchildren, 30% is provided by the spouse or partner, and only 4% comes from a person hired for the task. As for the people who provide help with instrumental activities, most come from sons, sons/daughters-in-law, or grandchildren (64%), about a third come from the spouse or partner, with a small fraction provided by paid caregivers (1%) (López-Ortega & Aranco, 2019).

1.3. Legislation

Although there are few legal precepts that can apply to LTC institutions, including temporary and permanent care for older people, no compulsory national level accreditation or standards of care are in place.

As one of its main attributions, INAPAM carries out inspection and surveillance visits to residential and care homes for older people in order to verify their operating conditions, training of their personnel, as well as quality of life of its residents. However, as a guideline for these supervision visits, INAPAM relies on the official Mexican standard "Social assistance services to adults and older people at risk and vulnerability" (NOM-SSA NOM-031-SSA3-2012, Asistencia Social. Prestación de Servicios de Asistencia Social a Adultos y Adultos Mayores en Situación de Riesgo y Vulnerabilidad), which only specifies basic safety and infrastructure requirements (e.g., ramps, handrails), recommends the type and number of professionals they should have (without taking into account total number of residents), and recommends basic care guidelines such as an annual medical evaluation for residents in institutions. Notably, this standard does not establish compulsory standards of care, outcome measures, care evaluation mechanisms, indicators to establish impact on resident's wellbeing, nor directives to enforce compliance.

With respect to legislation related to people with disabilities, Mexico has ratified international and inter-American treaties on disability, such as the Convention on the Rights of Persons with Disabilities (2008) and the Inter-American Convention for the Elimination of All Forms of Discrimination against People with Disabilities (1999). Within national legislation, the General Law for the Inclusion of People with Disabilities of 2011 lays the foundations for the full inclusion of people with disabilities, within a framework of equality in all areas of life. Notwithstanding the relevance of this Law, its focus is on achieving the integration of people with disabilities (formal education, workforce, recreational activities), and not on the need and obligation to provide direct care or support for people with disabilities or their family caregivers.

Regarding care legislation, there are no specific laws that guarantee the right to receive care, regardless of the age group or condition for which care is needed, or that give the health and social security system responsibility to provide them. As a consequence, public strategies to provide care and support for people with disabilities and care dependency and those who are currently caring for them are practically non-existent, and there is a clear lack of public programs at the national/ federal level that aim to provide care services for those with care needs, nor provide for their caregivers (Huenchuan-Navarro & Rodríguez-Velázquez, 2015; López-Ortega & Aranco, 2019).

2. Designing LTC Systems with a Systematic Approach

2.1. How Can We Apply a Systemic Approach to LTC Services in Mexico?

The focus on LTC has recently gained some attention in the academic and policy forums of Mexico, given the increasing awareness of the potential economic impacts from the demographic transition. As described earlier, the health and social sectors involved in solving the demand for LTC have been working separately, trying to solve their specific demands. Decision makers and ministries in Mexico have usually applied a vertical policy approach when trying to tackle a new issue. This means that new programs are created and implemented every time a new problem emerges. Programs emerge isolated from each other, with little connection among their goals and without efficient resource allocation, coordinated timing, or potential synergies among them. For example, although the current offer for LTC services in Mexico is diversified, it is fragmented and the maximum potential coverage is not reached because there might be overlapping services and poor integrative planning.

Literature about LTC has also changed from a programmatic (Muiser & Carrin, 2007; Swartz, 2013), to a more systemic approach (Villalobos Dintrans, 2018; Cafagna et al., 2019). A systemic approach to LTC in Mexico means:

1. Building a system to link the health and social sectors (and eventually the other sectors involved) by establishing systematic connections between them.
    - The LTC system is the connected set of all the resources efficiently shared between the health and social sectors to satisfy the demand of care services as a human right.
    - The LTC system will have three major connecting nodes for the health and social sectors to be linked: human capital, financing/infrastructure, and data and information.
2. Providing an integrative strategy to connect the currently isolated offer of LTC services in the country to enhance effectiveness and efficiency, as opposed to a programmatic, “vertical” response.

2.2. Rationale and Definition of the LTC System in Mexico

In the past, cultural factors were responsible for making the families fully responsible for the care needs of the individuals. Currently, middle-aged adults are experiencing pressure to simultaneously take care of their children and parents/grand-parents while at the same time, they are trying to pursue their professional goals. Also, with declining fertility rates, it is expected that the number of young adults "sustaining" the care burden of older people will decrease. In addition, increasing female leadership in many aspects of the professional environment is demanding new care options, rather than family-based ones (Lindt, van Berkel, & Mulder, 2020).

The Human Rights Chart and the Inter-American Convention on protecting the Human Rights of Older Persons (A-70) (Organization of American States, 2009) recognize health and care as human rights. As such, the State is responsible for providing the means for its satisfaction, and citizens are co-responsible in the process of making this a reality. On the other hand, the local constitution of Mexico City has recognized the right to care and the commitment of the State to implement a system for caregiving that offers quality public services (Administración Pública de la Ciudad de México, 2016).

Supported by these socio-cultural, demographic, and legal factors, an LTC system in Mexico is needed. Specifically, a system that can be more sustainable than the traditional scheme in which the amount of non-paid work related to care is 23.5% of the GDP (INEGI, 2018b). An integrated LTC system in Mexico could help to relieve the burden of Mexican families who struggle, or are not capable, to provide the care of their members. It is expected that an LTC system could also bring some economic benefits by allowing young adults (especially women) to have a more active participation in the labor market and the development of professional environments.

Table 2. Current institutional snapshot of LTC in Mexico

Sector	Institution	Funding	Area of interest	Target population
PUBLIC				
Ministry of well-being (social development)	INAPAM	100% allocations from public treasury	Healthy aging, daycare, professional training, cultural centers, among others	Older people
	DIF	100% allocations from public treasury	Violence, rehabilitation, nutritional assistance, attention to older people, among others	Families
	Universal pension	100% allocations from public treasury	Economic support	Older people
Ministry of Health	IMSS	Mixed: public funding and fees paid by the employers and employees	Healthy aging, medical and gerontological attention	Workers of the formal economy and their families
	ISSSTE	mixed: public funding and fees payed by the employers	Healthy aging, medical and gerontological attention	Older people beneficiaries of the institute
PRIVATE				
Non-profit organizations	Various	Donations, fees from beneficiaries	Nursing homes and day care centers	Poor and abandoned care-dependent older people
For profit organizations	Various	Investors and fees from the clients	Nursing homes/day care centers/ respite care	Care for dependent older people and their families

Source: Authors.

According to Colombo et al., (2011a),

> "LTC is the care for people needing support in many facets of living over a long period of time. Typically, this refers to help with so-called activities of daily living (ADL), such as bathing, dressing and getting out of bed, which are often performed by family, friends and lower-skilled caregivers or nurses."

We define the LTC system as the connected set of all the resources efficiently shared between the health and social sectors to satisfy the demand of services linked to care as a human right.

Colombo and colleagues' definition considers four components of an LTC system: beneficiaries, package of benefits, provider, and financing (Colombo, Llena-Nozal, Mercier, & Tjadens, 2011b). Our emphasis in this section will be on how some of these elements can serve as connecting nodes for the LTC system to be a system, rather than a pool of LTC services or programs.

2.3. Major Connecting Nodes of the LTC System

Systems are complex by definition. We recognize that creating an LTC system implies an enormous amount of effort, not only for its design but also for its implementation. Nevertheless, we think that there are three major connecting nodes that will be at the core of the linkage between the health, social, and other involved sectors: 1) human capital, 2) material capital (financing/infrastructure), and 3) meta-capital (data and information).

2.3.1. Human Capital

The current supply of care services for older people in Mexico is not systematically regulated. Many care homes and similar facilities have been operating for decades without proper certification obtained from either the health or social sectors. Therefore, the quality of the care delivered cannot be guaranteed and is not monitored by the government.

Training standards for caregivers should include knowledge, skills, abilities, and attitudes from the health and social domains; however, national level certification or standardized courses have recently become available. The National System of Proficiency and the National Council for the Standardization and Certification of Labor Proficiency (CONOCER, its acronym in Spanish), has developed proficiency standards for caregiving activities for older people both at home and in LTC facilities: "EC0665 - Care for the older people in permanent/temporary social assistance establishments" and "EC0669 - Basic care of the older person at home." Recently, the National Institute of Geriatrics (INGER) was accredited as a Centre for proficiency certification and Evaluation. In 2017, INGER founded and currently chairs the Geriatrics Proficiency Committee. This committee has developed several proficiency standards related to health care and social care for the older people, including:

- "EC1209 - Providing guidance support to informal caregivers of the older people,"
- "EC0964 - Assessment of the functional ability of older people"
- "EC0965 - Management of risk factors for disability in older people"
- "EC1141 - Application of individualized programs of multicomponent physical activity for older people"
- "EC1142 - Nutritional orientation for older people"
- "EC1208 - Application of an individual program of cognitive stimulation for older people"

Another proficiency standard of care for care dependent older people is currently under development. The proficiency standards are published in the official gazette of the federation and provide reference for the design of training and certification programs within the Ministry of Public Education.

The Education and Outreach Direction of INGER has been conducting training and certification for three years. This duty is foreseen to be scaled-up nationwide to improve the performance of the caregivers for older people.

An increasing demand for care services brings an opportunity to activate the labor market. The health and social sectors should decide to invest in human capital because, as explained earlier, families will not be able to sustain caregiving as they currently do. Also, opening positions for caregivers with proper labor conditions inside the public or private systems will help to activate the economy and have a positive impact on the development of the country. For this to happen within the public sector, specific "profiles" need to be created, because the current structure does not include the profile for caregivers or even gerontologists. This means that they are not eligible for a formal contract inside the health system in Mexico.

2.3.1.1. How Is This Strategy Going To Connect The Involved Sectors?

Both the health and the social sectors should suggest contents for the strategy for human resources capacity building. For example, primary healthcare personnel as well as those working in hospitals and institutionalized settings should receive updated information about the way the LTC system is expected to work, and the role each one plays in order to maintain the connectivity of caregiving pathways. Enhancing technology-based communication will be fundamental for the success of the caregiving team (CT) (see below, section "Meta-Capital").

Continuous education for medical and non-medical staff should allow all members of the CT to "speak the same language," for instance, interpreting the scores of functional outcomes and the usage of frequently used terms such as "frailty" or "caregiver burnout."

Also, the education and labor sectors should recognize the validity of the programs and provide (education) and request (labor) a certificate for the people willing to work as caregivers.

2.3.1.2. The Role of Gerontologists

Two approaches to gerontology supplement each other in Mexico: the empirical-positivist branch, with a focus on measuring biomedical and social variables in older people; and the theoretical-critical branch, focused on the study of the aging process from the sociological point of view. Usually, programs for gerontologist training are biased toward one or the other branch, according to the expertise of the professors.

Consensus is needed regarding the core knowledge and skills required in gerontology training. Envisioning the gerontologist as a case manager could provide insight for reaching such consensus. In the context of fragmented health and social security systems in Mexico, gerontologists could be very helpful to guide those needing care and their families as they "navigate" through pathways of care.

The gerontologists can be the element of the LTC system closest to those needing care. They could decide the best entry point to the system every time an older person asks for help. For example, if help is requested because of an episode of acute pain, the gerontologist could take a look at the personal health record and individualized care plan of the person and decide what could be the best approach.

2.3.1.3. Designing Person-Centered Care Plans

Individualized care plans, established with an integrative approach by the CT, will dictate the goals and the expected time to reach milestones, as well as organize the role of each member of the CT to avoid duplicated efforts and reduce omissions.

Integrated Care for Older People (ICOPE) launched by the World Health Organization (WHO) (World Health Organization, 2019) includes a model of care that can be adapted to the Mexican local context. ICOPE provides guidance to design and implement individualized care plans, along with others like the Strengthening Responses to Dementia in Developing Countries (STRiDE) project.

The idea is that after an initial assessment, the CT can gather to discuss the patient's case and design a care plan. The goals and milestones of the care plan can be uploaded to the patient's electronic health record, reachable by anyone in the CT, including the patient. For example, if a patient arrives at the hospital for an acute problem, the medical staff can access his/her care plan and may choose to provide a solution in the ER, rather than hospitalizing him/her. Any adjustments to the care plan could be updated in real time using the LTC virtual platform (See below, section "Meta-Capital").

2.3.2. Material Capital: Financing Alternatives for the LTC System

Financing is another dimension revealing the systemic nature of the LTC issue, because the mechanisms to finance LTC systems are closely linked to the resources of the health care and pension systems. In Figure 1 we represent this idea like three chained elephants. If one of them moves, it will inevitably cause the other two to move, and all of them will be fighting to move in their desired direction. This could happen especially if the three elephants share the same funding source.

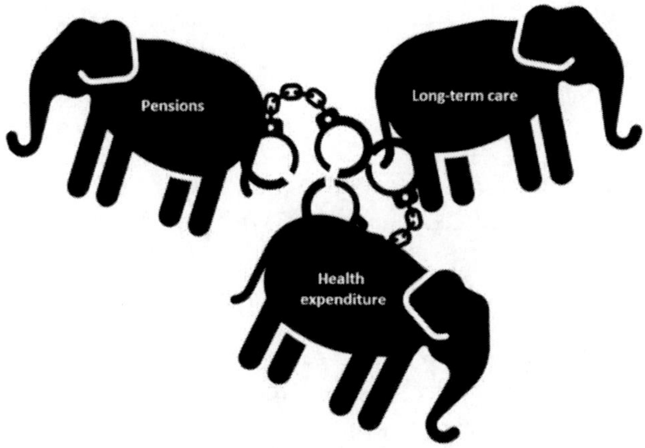

Source: Image adapted from personal communications between Emmanuel Gonzalez, Enrique Vega and Pablo Villalobos Dintrans.

Figure 1. Tax-based financing sources for LTC: the three chained elephants.

An LTC system can help by bringing balance to the interplay between pensions, health expenditures, and financing sources for LTC.

Is LTC social insurance the best way of financing the LTC system in Mexico? We consider that the social insurance scheme could be feasible for a segment of the employees with upper-middle to high incomes; this group is currently a minority (INEGI, 2018a). A national fund for LTC could be pooled from the contributions of the employees and employers. This type of scheme has the advantage that it allows prediction of the amount of resources available, since there is a specific fund, but it would be less flexible in terms of the benefits because those would need to be fixed a priori. For example, an employee who experienced dementia at age 85 might not be covered by social security insurance for 24-hour caregiving in a nursing home if this was not included in his contract when he started working at 33. Moreover, given that wages in Mexico are among the lowest in Latin America, a careful evaluation of how mandatory contributions for social insurance could affect household income is needed.

Therefore, tax-based financing could be an alternative financing scheme for the majority of the population who live and work outside of the formal sector, but who make high contributions to the economy via care-related non-paid work. A pre-requisite for going forward in this direction is to evaluate the costs of not having the system and continuing business as usual versus the potential costs and investment needed to build the LTC system.

According to González-González et al., (2019), an LTC system in Mexico would cost between 0.17% and 0.45% of the GDP in 2026. This estimation is based on population projections for people aged 60 years and older who reported difficulty with at least one of the ADLs. It includes 50% coverage for people with severe dependence: 120 hours/month for personal in-home assistants, tele-assistance technology, one monthly medical consultation; 10% coverage for LTC residences; and 25% coverage for people with mild dependence: 20 hours/month for personal in-home assistants and tele-assistance technology. We think this is a very conservative estimation because of the low coverage levels and the exclusion of day-care and services for the caregiver.

On the other hand, not having an LTC system in Mexico also entails costs, starting with the fact that up to 23.3% of older people with some ADL difficulty would be lacking any type of care.

The indirect costs of not having an LTC system in place include: the cost of health care derived from physical and psychological problems in caregivers, their reduced participation in the labor market, and increasing out-of-pocket health payments by caregivers in households with older people (Pan American Health Organization, 2019). For example, in Chile, the estimated costs of not having an LTC system range between US$ 698 million and 19.6 billion per year, depending on the definitions and packages of services included (Villalobos Dintrans, 2018).

It is not our aim to extensively review the alternative financing schemes for the LTC system that could work in Mexico, but our perspective is that the most suitable scheme considered so far would be a mixed one: it could be predominantly based on tax revenues, with a lower proportion based on social security, the private sector, and out-of-pocket payments. It would be useful to estimate the cost-effectiveness threshold for this scheme using another marker, such as the Activities of Daily Living Adjusted Year (ADLAY) that is, the amount of money needed to gain one year of life of having basic ADLs needs improved, from these needs being entirely unmet to being fully met(Wittenberg & Malley, 2007).

2.3.2.1. Existing Infrastructure and New Infrastructure That Is Needed

Cash transfers have been a predominant strategy of the current Mexican government to implement social policy. Although cash transfers have had a positive impact in some specific cases (Salinas-Rodríguez, Torres-Pereda, Manrique-Espinoza, Moreno-Tamayo, & Téllez-Rojo Solís, 2014), they fail to achieve social development if not accompanied by the creation of infrastructure. Building facilities adapted for disabled users' needs is important. Even if up to 90% of dependent older people are non-institutionalized currently, nursing homes represent a solution for the severely disabled, highly isolated population, and for those at high risk of domestic violence. The question is: what kind of nursing homes? Can innovation make nursing homes fit in the so-called "community-based" and "person-centered" LTC facilities? One example of this could be the "Green House® Project" in the United States, which uses the approach of clusters of small houses (with 6-10 older people living in independent rooms, but with access to common spaces), surrounded by natural open spaces (The Green House Project, 2020).

Care homes should have a link to community life (while maintaining resident safety). Imagine, for example, that there is a playground installed in the garden of a nursing home, and children may come and play. This might reduce social isolation of the residents and is also beneficial for their health (Liu et al., 2020). Flexible arrangements for LTC facilities would allow them to adapt to the different kinds of services needed, which would be 80% social services and 20% health services, on average.

The systemic approach of a community-based LTC system considers territorial networks as functional units including private housing, nursing homes, a community clinic, and a reference hospital within a reasonable distance, ideally reachable by public transportation. This approach has not been used in Mexico before, but other countries have applied it. One example is the integrated community care system in Japan (Sakamoto et al., 2018). We think that having a geocoded map of LTC offerings and using the territorial networks approach (rather than political divisions) can be helpful to policy makers to identify territories (cities/towns) with an urgent coverage gap. Also, this map could be a tool for families of older people in need of care and case managers to find the most optimal LTC offer available.

2.3.3. Meta-Capital/Information System

LTC systems need other kind of intangible resources: data and information systems. Technological resources will be crucial to providing close communication and stronger therapeutic relationships across professional boundaries among the members of the CT, which will empower the patients and benefit their outcomes. Also, technology and innovation can help by creating networks and communities to support patients (Collins, 2020). Examples of this include the creation of a National Registry of Caregiving and the LTC virtual platform, which would enable the flow of data between the care recipients, their case managers, and other members of the CT. This is still an aspirational aspect of LTC in Mexico, and potential drawbacks of its implementation should be tackled by an interdisciplinary team.

2.4. Implementation Route Map: Who, What, to Whom, and How?

Recently, INGER hosted the APEC collaborative workshop "Capacity building for community-based LTC." Participants from the Asia-Pacific region and the Americas shared the state-of-the-art in LTC. Academic experts provided useful insight about designing and implementing LTC systems in developing countries. Based on the lessons learned during the workshop and on previous work from INGER experts, we have determined the following elements to be helpful in guiding the design and implementation of an LTC system in Mexico (Instituto Nacional de Geriatría, 2020a).

- LTC network: institutionalization of the cluster of stakeholders at national and local levels
- The model of care and the warranted package of core interventions: we envision a model of integrated care for older people adapted from the ICOPE proposal of the WHO
- Profile of the potential recipients of LTC services
- Settings for the delivery of LTC services
- Challenges and opportunities derived from the COVID-19 pandemic for Mexican LTC services.

3. Characteristics and Preparedness of LTC Institutions in Mexico: The Example of the COVID-19 Pandemic

The 2019 coronavirus disease (COVID-19) pandemic during the first months of 2020 dramatically affected LTC facilities (LTCF) in several European countries, with around 40% of COVID-19 deaths occurring in LTCF residents (World Health Organization, 2020). When the pandemic reached the Americas, affecting the United States and Canada, a large part of COVID-19 fatalities occurred in LTCF (Yourish, Rebeca, Ivory, & Smith, 2020).

The situation in Mexico may have not been as acute, given the small proportion of older people living in LTCF (less than 1%): the vast majority live in their homes (Instituto Nacional de Geografía y Estadística, 2015). However, the press informed the public of some outbreaks that occurred in LTCF in various states in the country, such as Nuevo León (Redacción, 2020c), Tabasco (Redacción, 2020a), Tamaulipas (Sanchéz & Chio, 2020), Baja California (Redacción, 2020b), Morelos (Tonantzin, 2020), Chihuahua (Estrada, 2020), Mexico City (Becerril & Wong, 2020), and Coahuila (Redacción, 2020d), among others.

INAPAM, the government entity with the legal responsibility for supervising LTCF, published a contingency operating protocol for gerontological centers with permanent residents, in light of the epidemiological alert for COVID-19 (Instituto Nacional de las Personas Adultas Mayores, 2020b). This protocol recommended LTCFs take action to prevent and manage COVID-19 outbreaks by incorporating INGER guidelines. The protocol was disseminated to several LTCF through the communication and training areas of the Private Assistance Board of Mexico City and other similar organizations.

The public sector has exercised several actions towards the containment and prevention of COVID-19 in residents of LTCF. However, these actions have been only informative, for the most part. Except for some interventions at the local government level, there was no direct linkage with active epidemiological surveillance services and no specific actions were in place in order to detect asymptomatic and pre-symptomatic cases, nor was there a link to public medical care services for suspected or confirmed cases of COVID-19. These actions were also insufficient to guarantee timely and effective care, nor did they allow for the provision of palliative care in severe cases or for people with advance directives that established their preference for no hospitalization and no invasive mechanical ventilation, but did specify relief of suffering, associated with dyspnea, pain or other symptoms of the disease.

The COVID-19 pandemic evidenced the lags in LTC that have existed in Mexico for decades; the poor quality of services provided in this type of institution in the public, social, and private sectors had been documented (Comisión de Derechos Humanos del Distrito Federal, 2008; Gutiérrez-Robledo, Reyes-Ortega, Rocabado-Quevedo, & López-Franchini, 1996). However, efforts had been made in this area in recent years: the agreement of the highest authority of the health sector in Mexico to lay the foundations for the creation of a National LTC System (Consejo de Salubridad General, 2018); the development of a proposal that guides the design of public policy with emphasis on the community component of this type of services (Instituto Nacional de Geriatría, 2019); the preparation of a project to update the official Mexican standard that regulates the LCTF in the country (Secretaría de Salud, 2019); and the incorporation of this issue as a priority objective of the sectoral program of the Ministry of Welfare at the federal level (Secretaría de Bienestar, 2020).

While these are steps that will allow moving forward, there are still many challenges to face in order to achieve the effective implementation of a national LTC system in Mexico. This includes the urgent improvement of the quality of services provided in LTCF, through the professionalization of the personnel who work in them, the establishment of quality standards, the creation of an information system, and the link between social and health services. In addition, there are indispensable fiscal reforms and other components of responsibilities of the State and society as contemplated in the LTC axis of the World Health Organization's global strategy and action plan for the decade of healthy aging 2020-2030 (World Health Organization, 2017).

National Institute of Geriatrics of Mexico and the mitigation of the COVID-19 pandemic in Mexican long-term care facilities.

Faced with the tragic situation that occurred in nursing homes during the COVID-19 pandemic in countries such as Italy, Spain, the United Kingdom, the United States and Canada (World Health Organization, 2020), since the end of March 2020, INGER undertook the task of generating information regarding the degree of preparedness of LTCF in the country to face the pandemic and minimize its impact in terms of infections and deaths in Mexico.

INGER published a COVID-19 prevention guide for older people's residences (Instituto Nacional de Geriatría, 2020d) based on the recommendations issued in countries that had already suffered outbreaks of infection of severe acute respiratory syndrome type 2 coronavirus (SARS-CoV-2) in their LTCF Simultaneously, we started a survey (Instituto Nacional de Geriatría, 2020c) to determine how prepared LTCF were to prevent and manage outbreaks of COVID-19. This allowed for the identification of a greater number of residences than those officially registered in the existing information systems at the time.

4. Next Steps for the LTC System in Mexico

We propose three pillars for the National LTC System in Mexico: 1) the National Care System Council comprising relevant stakeholders[1], 2) a decision-making platform, and 3) an integrated information system. This would not require the creation of new institutions. The principles that should govern the LTC strategy in Mexico are: a human rights approach; solidarity (resources are distributed); universality (resources are distributed to the entire population that meets the requirements and has a need for care); and progressiveness (the system must first provide for the needs of populations with lower access to resources and public services). On the other hand, there are still unsolved issues, like defining the specific roles of each stakeholder and clear standard procedures of how to manage the financial and other resources.

[1] Ministries of Wellbeing and Social Development, Health, Work, and Education; social security institutes; DIF family development system; and civil society organizations and institutions with related mandates in cross-cutting areas, such as The Institute for Women (INMUJERES) and the Council for prevention of discrimination (CONAPRED).

4.1. Transformation of Cultural and Organizational Structures

Advancing toward the LTC system for Mexico requires changes both at the social mindset and organizational levels (Figure 2):

- Changing the perception of LTC as a charity-based activity or an exclusive responsibility of the family to the paradigm of LTC as a right
- Placing LTC at the top of the public agenda
- Decrease the burden on families and help the caregivers
- Recognize the social value of caregivers, who should receive compensation and social acknowledgement for the tasks performed

First, programs should prioritize and facilitate safe and patient-centered in-home primary and acute care and long-term services and support (LTSS) delivery. Individuals should have freedom of choice as to how and where they receive care. As most older people prefer to live at home as they age, the best care models will be the ones that allow them to stay in their preferred environment, where they are stimulated mentally and physically and are comfortable. Traditional care models resign older people to care facilities, but as they strive and can stay independent for longer, they should have options for where they live and receive their care. Care for older people must be about much more than accomplishing tasks; it should be personal and personalized, based on validated instruments that assess the needs and wants of older individuals. By identifying these needs, caregivers and society at large can better and more compassionately respond and keep older people engaged and safe from neglect. As society has accepted the ethical responsibility to care for the young, we too must commit to care for the old.

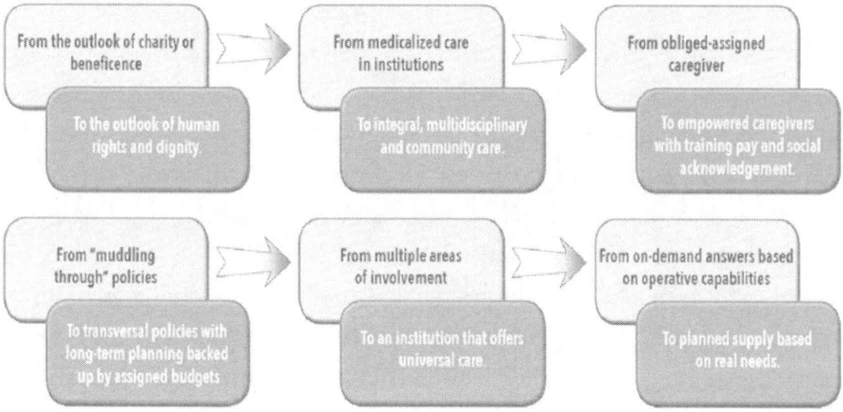

Source: Instituto Nacional de Geriatría. (2019). [Diagnosis and proposal: long-term care at the community level in Mexico]. Diagnóstico y propuesta: cuidados a largo plazo a nivel comunitario en México (1st ed.). Mexico City: INGER.

Figure 2. Transformation of the current structures and paradigms.

4.2. 21st-Century Care Models Should Meet 21st-Century Quality Expectations

Care services should be delivered responsibly, with the highest ethical standards, personal regard for older people and their families, and utmost attention to health, home, and personal care. Therefore, whether care is provided by government services, charitable organizations, or the private sector, we must expect of ourselves and others that caregivers are well trained and compassionate. Caregiving and quality standards are to be developed within COFEPRIS and the National Public Health Council.

4.3. Caregivers Play a Critical Role in Health and Prevention

Caregivers are the lynchpin for restoring and maintaining the health of older people. Competency standards developed for them must be generalized. Special attention must be paid to preserve intrinsic capacity, paying attention to its domains as well as to non-communicable diseases

(NCDs) that are common with age, including Alzheimer's disease, cardiovascular disease, and diabetes. The deterioration of mobility, loss of vision, hearing, bone, and muscle mass affect quality of life, have an impact on falls, and can lead to other age-related health risks. Providing care that anticipates and provides for these conditions will keep older people healthier and can reduce system-wide health care costs. The ICOPE strategy is essential to these aims (WHO, 2018).

Policymakers should address social risk, through enhanced virtual supports and bridging of the digital divide. Technology can enable efficiency of care. Although beneficial for tele-health, social interactions, and increasing access to vital medical and social resources, information and communication technologies (ICTs) remain inaccessible to many older people in Mexico, due to resources, information, or usability constraints. Technology has a critical role to play in monitoring the health of older people and keeping them connected in society. Technology cannot replace the human touch when it comes to personalized care, but it can make the care process more efficient and coordinated. The right balance between the two is essential to ensure 21st-century care needs are met with 21st-century care solutions.

4.4. Care Is Linked to Family Structure

Family dynamics are changing in light of the fact that there will soon be more "old" than "young." The demands on family caregivers are increasing, as they balance employment and caregiving responsibilities and often neglect their own health. By supplementing family caregiving with high-quality, reliable, and compassionate models of care, the physical and emotional burdens on families can be alleviated and the family structure restored. Additionally, intergenerational programming should be broadly incorporated into LTC. The massive expansion of in-home health and LTC required to address the pandemic's disability cascade can benefit from intergenerational service. Intergenerational programs provide bidirectional benefits and are popular: they can involve younger individuals, who provide companionship to older people and offer caregivers respite, as well as older people's volunteerism, which improves cognition and functioning and younger adult educational performance and attitudes and behaviors toward aging and older people.

4.5. Caregiving can be a Path to Economic Growth and Job Creation

Caregiving is relational and reciprocal. It can be thought of, in an anthropological sense, as a gift exchange. In this moral, emotional, and practical exchange, the gift of the person's human need for assistance to reduce pain and alleviate suffering and her responses to the care provided is reciprocated by the return gift of acknowledging, affirming, and responding in equally human ways (Kleinman, 2015). But caregiving as a profession also presents opportunities for new jobs, productivity, and economic growth. With a shortage of family caregivers as a result of more old than young people, a trend which is global and growing, we need to view caregiving as an opportunity to meet the following societal and economic goals:

- To keep family caregivers healthy and therefore more productive in the workforce and in society;
- To engage older people so they may stay as active as possible—physically, mentally, socially—for as long as possible;
- To provide jobs for individuals with the skills and compassion to provide care for elders;
- To provide training and skills for individuals entering one of the many professions within the care field; and
- To define a growing and transformative profession that will be relevant and essential for generations to come.

4.6. Building an Aging-Friendly Physical and Social Infrastructure

Aging-friendly physical and social infrastructures should be implemented to promote supportive, socially cohesive communities. Many communities require additional external supports to develop age-friendly environments, even as social capital and cohesion may naturally form in others during times of crisis. Supports from trusted organizations that work and interact with community dwelling older people on a regular basis (e. g. day centers) can help connect supply with demand, as can social media platforms. Such interventions can lead to the development of social capital and cohesion within communities that have lasting impact beyond the pandemic.

4.7. Pending Tasks to Advance the Design and Implementation of an LTC System in Mexico

Research:

- Define the current and projected demand for services
  - Derived from the estimation and projection of the functional dependence of older people and the costs associated with this, both for health services and households, including an estimate of the financial, human, and infrastructure resources needed to operate a system
- Obtain funding for research studies
  - Preferences of beneficiaries and their caregivers and the types of supports needed: monetary, respite care, day centers, others. This should be done before generating specific household support strategies, as it is critical to know what would be acceptable and what would not, to prevent failed programs
  - In-depth study of the costs associated with care and the effects of care dependency

  - Improvements in population levels of intrinsic capacity and functional ability to prevent/postpone care dependency.

Care provision:

- Obtain commitment from the Ministry of Health and the Ministry of Wellbeing
  - For the provision of LTC services, including health and social services, as well as for the regulation of ongoing institutions. All this under a multidimensional and cross-sectorial integration perspective
  - The sector program of the Ministry of Welfare 2020-2024, contemplates as part of its priority objectives the implementation of a national care system; similarly, the sector program of the Ministry of Health 2020-2024 includes as a priority strategy to strengthen a model of comprehensive care and social assistance to optimize the efficiency and effectiveness of the processes and expand the coverage of health services and social assistance
- Generate multidimensional strategies
  - Support for family members or primary caregivers to reduce the direct and indirect costs generated by the care they perform, including accompaniment and support services in personal care activities
  - Extend home health visit models for dependent older people
  - Respite centers for family caregivers
  - Generate LTC models within the framework of primary health care

More explicit regulatory framework:

- The National commission for prevention of sanitary risks and the National Public Health Council should function together as the regulatory entity for the LTC system, in charge of supervising, evaluating and, where appropriate, punishing those that do not comply.

- The General Public Health Council should promote the declaration of enforceability governing the provision of LTC so that the Ministry of Health can propose the relevant official standard, as well as a national training program
- Establish a mandatory national registry to which all LTC institutions must register, regardless of their nature or financing condition, in order to specify control and surveillance actions towards these establishments, while having a publicly accessible information tool for all potential users of these institutions and their families
- The regulations relating to social assistance (Official Mexican Standard NOM-031-SSA3-2012, and its proposed update Project of Official Mexican Standard PROY-NOM-031-SSA3-2018), which refer mainly to vulnerable populations that include older people, are insufficient as a regulatory instrument of LTC institutions for older people

- Develop the requirements under which LTC institutions will be permitted to operate (mandatory quality standards of national enforcement)
- Develop an accreditation program for both LTC institutions and staff, in equivalence to the certification program for health service providers

4.8. Reimagining Long-Term Care

"Caregiving is a defining condition of what it means to be human. Its scope is broad and encompasses care of children, care of the sick, care of older people or those who live with disabilities, and care of the dying" (Kleinman, 2015). This view is a neglected aspect of policy making in the field. The eloquent plea by Arthur Kleinman for caregiving to be viewed as an important and positive aspect of life and medicine still demands serious attention, five years after its publication. It also requires a substantive shift in attitudes and language on the parts of both policy makers and health-care professionals. All too often, care of those affected by illness and disability, particularly in later life, is portrayed in terms of burden.

The caregiver burden has become a dominant topic both in the study and in the practical approach to the state of caring. As caregivers, we refuse this simplistic characterization. People are willing to care for their vulnerable relatives, but they need assistance to ease the burdensome aspects of care as much as possible through solidarity, information, and support. We need to find a language and processes that reflect this complexity, and to draw more from the small but growing scientific literature on the positive aspects of caregiving, so as to help with an aspect of life that reflects both our existential vulnerability and our mutual interdependence.

The COVID-19 public health emergency has introduced new threats to LTC systems. Novel approaches to establish supports and services are required to supplement ruptured formal and informal caregiving and social interactions. We need an innovative care intervention framework that relies on reimagined clinical and community supports, involving links with in-home primary care, massive dissemination of tele-health technology, support for vulnerable older people, and intergenerational exchanges. Together, with support from local and national organizations supporting aging, these policies can rebuild resilient, aging-friendly communities and structures and promote a sense of societal cohesion.

Take home messages:

- Learning from the experiences of other countries has been enlightening to begin the drafting of the most feasible model for LTC in Mexico.
- It is important and necessary to achieve a multiparty regulatory entity to provide and evaluate the standards of technical requirements and quality LTC services.
- The National Institute of Geriatrics should take advantage of the extraordinary opportunity and momentum to advocate for the

alignment and integration of the existing institutions toward an LTC system in Mexico.

References

Administración Pública de la Ciudad de México. (2016). *Constitución Política de la Ciudad de México*. Retrieved from http://www.infodf.org.mx/documentospdf/constitucion_cdmx/Constitucion_Politica_CDMX.pdf. [Public Administration of Mexico City. (2016). *Political Constitution of Mexico City*.]

Becerril, J., & Wong, A. P. (2020, May 25). [*Nursing home evicted in the municipality of Cuauhtémoc due to coronavirus outbreak*]. Desalojan asilo en la alcaldía Cuauhtémoc por brote de coronavirus. Milenio. Retrieved from https://www.milenio.com/politica/comunidad/coronavirus-cdmx-desaloja-asilo-casos-covid-19.

Cafagna, G., Aranco, N., Ibarrarán, P., Oliveri, M. L., Medellín, N., & Stampini, M. (2019). *Age with Care*. Washington, D.C.

Collins, B. (2020). *Technology and innovation for long-term health conditions|The King's Fund*. Retrieved from https://www.kingsfund.org.uk/publications/technology-innovation-long-term-health-conditions.

Colombo, F., Llena-Nozal, A., Mercier, J., & Tjadens, F. (2011a). *Help Wanted?* https://doi.org/10.1787/9789264097759-en.

Colombo, F., Llena-Nozal, A., Mercier, J., & Tjadens, F. (2011b). Long-term Care: Growing Sector, Multifaceted Systems. *Help Wanted? Providing and Paying for Long-Term Care*, 37–60. https://doi.org/10.1787/9789264097759-en.

Comisión de Derechos Humanos del Distrito Federal. (2008). *Informe especial sobre la situación de los derechos humanos de las personas adultas mayores en las instituciones del Distrito Federal*. 2007. Retrieved from www.cdhdf.org.mx. [*Special report on the situation of human rights of older persons in the institutions of the Federal District*]

Consejo de Salubridad General, P. (2018, August 2). [*Agreement establishing the actions for the design and implementation of the public health policy for the granting of long-term care by public institutions of the National Health System*] Acuerdo por el que se establecen las acciones para el diseño e imple. *Diario Oficial de La Federación.* Retrieved from http://www.dof.gob.mx/nota_detalle.php?codigo=5533729&fecha=02/08/2018.

Díaz-Venegas, C., De La Vega, S., & Wong, R. (2015). Transitions in activities of daily living in Mexico, 2001-2012. *Salud Publica de Mexico, 57 Suppl 1*(0 1), S54-61. https://doi.org/10.21149/spm.v57s1.7590.

DIF - Transparencia DIF Nacional. (2020, January 17). *Centros Gerontológicos.* Retrieved October 13, 2020, from http://sitios.dif.gob.mx/transparencia/transparencia_focalizada/centros_gerontologicos/centros_gerontologicos.html. [*Gerontological Centers.*]

Estrada, J. (2020, August 30). [*Covid-19 outbreak denounced in Chihuahua nursing home*]. Denuncian brote de Covid-19 en asilo de Chihuahua. La Jornada. Retrieved from https://www.jornada.com.mx/ultimas/estados/2020/05/12/denuncian-brote-de-covid-19-en-asilo-de-chihuahua-3971.html.

García-Peña, C., Ávila-Funes, J. A., Dent, E., Gutiérrez-Robledo, L., & Pérez-Zepeda, M. (2016). Frailty prevalence and associated factors in the Mexican health and aging study: A comparison of the frailty index and the phenotype. *Experimental Gerontology*, *79*, 55–60. https://doi.org/10.1016/j.exger.2016.03.016.

González-González, C., Stampini, M., Cafagna, G., Hernández Ruiz, M. del C., & Ibarrarán, P. (2019). Simulaciones del costo de un sistema de apoyo para los adultos mayores en situación de dependencia en México. In *Documento de Trabajo.* [Simulations of the cost of a support system for dependent older adults in Mexico. In *Working Document*]

Gutiérrez Robledo, L. M., López Ortega, M., & Arango Lopera, V. E. (2012). The State of Elder Care in Mexico. *Current Geriatrics Reports*, *1*(4), 183–189. https://doi.org/10.1007/s13670-012-0028-z.

Gutiérrez-Robledo, L. M., Reyes-Ortega, G., Rocabado-Quevedo, F., & López-Franchini, J. (1996). [Studies in the Federal District on the microbial content of some food from meat and its application in the control of the same]. Evaluación de instituciones de cuidados prolongados para ancianos en el Distrito Federal. Una visión crítica. *Salud Publica de Mexico*, *38*(6), 487–500. Retrieved from https://pubmed.ncbi.nlm.nih.gov/9054018/.

Huenchuan Navarro, S., & Rodríguez Velázquez, R. I. (2015). *Necesidades de cuidado de las personas mayores en la Ciudad de México: diagnóstico y lineamientos de política* (No. 664). Retrieved from CEPAL website: https://repositorio.cepal.org//handle/11362/38879. [*Elderly care needs in Mexico City: diagnosis and policy guidelines*]

INEGI. (2014). Directorio Nacional de Unidades Económicas. DENUE. *Censos Económicos 2014*. Retrieved from https://www.inegi.org.mx/app/mapa/denue/.

INEGI. (2015). *Censo de Alojamientos de Asistencia Social 2015*. Retrieved from https://www.inegi.org.mx/programas/caas/2015/. [*Census of Social Assistance Accommodation 2015*.]

INEGI. (2018a). *Encuesta Nacional de Ingresos y Gastos de los Hogares (ENIGH). 2018 Nueva serie*. Retrieved October 12, 2020, from https://www.inegi.org.mx/programas/enigh/nc/2018/default.html#Tabulados. [*National Survey of Household Income and Expenditure (ENIGH). 2018 New series*]

INEGI. (2018b). *Trabajo No Remunerado de los Hogares*. Base 2013. Retrieved August 7, 2020, from Sistema de Cuentas Nacionales de México. website: https://www.inegi.org.mx/temas/tnrh/. [*Unpaid Household Work*]

Instituto Nacional de Estadística y Geografía. (2015, December 8). *Resultados Definitivos De La Encuesta Intercensal 2015* (pp. 1–4). pp. 1–4. Retrieved from https://www.inegi.org.mx/contenidos/programas/intercensal/2015/doc/especiales2015_12_3.pdf. [*Final Results of the Intercensal Survey 2015*]

Instituto Nacional de Geografía y Estadística, P. (2015). [*Census of Social Assistance Housing 2015*]. Censo de Alojamientos de Asistencia

Social 2015. Retrieved August 16, 2020, from INEGI website: https://www.inegi.org.mx/programas/caas/2015/default.html# Tabulados.

Instituto Nacional de Geriatría, P. (2019). [*Diagnosis and proposal: long-term care at the community level in Mexico*]. *Diagnóstico y propuesta: cuidados a largo plazo a nivel comunitario en México* (1st ed.). Mexico City: INGER.

Instituto Nacional de Geriatría, P. (2020c). [*Measurement and Monitoring of the Preparation and Local Response to the COVID-19 Pandemic in Long-Term Care Facilities in Mexico*]. *Medición y Seguimiento de la Preparación y Respuesta Local a la Pandemia de COVID-19 en Instituciones de Cuidados a Largo P.* Retrieved August 16, 2020, from http://www.geriatria.salud.gob.mx/contenidos/institucional/medicion-seguimiento-instituciones-residencias-covid.html.

Instituto Nacional de Geriatría, P. (2020d). [*Prevention of coronavirus disease 2019 in residences for older people*]. *Prevención de enfermedad por coronavirus 2019 en residencias de personas mayores.* Retrieved August 16, 2020, from INGER website: http://www. geriatria.salud.gob.mx/contenidos/institucional/prevencion-enfermedad-personas-mayores.html.

Instituto Nacional de Geriatría. (2020a). *Capacity Building For Community-Based Long-Term Care.* Retrieved October 13, 2020, from Workshop report website: http://geriatria.salud.gob.mx/contenidos/institucional/taller-apec-inger-clp-comunitarios.html.

Instituto Nacional de Geriatría. (2020b). *Envejecimiento y dependencia: Retos y propuestas para la investigación en políticas públicas basadas en evidencia.* Mexico City: INGER. [*Aging and dependency: Challenges and proposals for evidence-based public policy research*.]

Instituto Nacional de las Personas Adultas Mayores, P. (2020b). [*Contingency operating protocol in gerontological centers of permanent stay due to the epidemiological alert for coronavirus (COVID-19)*]. *Protocolo operativo de contingencia en centros gerontológicos de estancia permanente por la alerta epidemiológica por.*

Instituto Nacional de las Personas Adultas Mayores. (2020a, March 12). *Albergues y Residencias de día INAPAM*. Retrieved October 13, 2020, from https://www.gob.mx/inapam/acciones-y-programas/albergues-y-residencias-diurnas-inapam. [*INAPAM Day Hostels and Residences*]

Kleinman, A. (2015, July 18). Care: In search of a health agenda. *The Lancet*, Vol. 386, pp. 240–241. https://doi.org/10.1016/S0140-6736(15)61271-5.

Lindt, N., van Berkel, J., & Mulder, B. C. (2020). Determinants of overburdening among informal carers: a systematic review. *BMC Geriatrics*, *20*(1), 304. https://doi.org/10.1186/s12877-020-01708-3.

Liu, C. C., Sun, Y., Kung, S. F., Kuo, H. W., Huang, N. C., Li, C. Y., & Hu, S. C. (2020). Effects of physical and social environments on the risk of dementia among Taiwanese older people: a population-based case-control study. *BMC Geriatrics*, *20*(1), 226. https://doi.org/10.1186/s12877-020-01624-6.

López-Ortega, M. (2018). *Cuidados de la Salud de los Adultos Mayores. Suplemento TODAS.* Mexico City: INMUJERES. [*Health Care of the Elderly. ALL supplement.*]

López-Ortega, M., & Aranco, N. (2019). *Envejecimiento y atención a la dependencia en México*. https://doi.org/10.18235/0001826. [*Aging and care for dependency in Mexico*.]

López-Ortega, M., & Jiménez-Bolón, J. (2015). Dependencia y Cuidados de Largo Plazo. In L. Gutiérrez Robledo, M. García Peña, & J. Jiménez Bolón (Eds.), *Envejecimiento Y Dependencia Realidades Y Previsión Para Los Próximos Años.* Retrieved from https://www.anmm.org.mx/publicaciones/CAnivANM150/L11-Envejecimiento-y-dependencia.pdf. [Dependency and Long Term Care. In L. Gutiérrez Robledo, M. García Peña, & J. Jiménez Bolón (Eds.), *Aging and Dependence Realities and Forecast for the Coming Years*]

Muiser, J., & Carrin, G. (2007). *Financing long-term care programmes in health systems with a situation assessment in selected.* Retrieved from https://www.who.int/health_financing/documents/dp_e_07_6-longtermcare.pdf?ua=1.

Organization of American States: (2009, August 1). *Inter-American Convention On Protecting The Human Rights Of Older Persons* (A-70). *2020*.

Pan American Health Organization. (2019). *Long-term care in the Americas*.

Redacción. (2020a, May 7). [One older adult died and 5 serious due to outbreaks in nursing homes in Tabasco and NL]. Un adulto mayor fallecido y 5 graves por brotes de COVID-19 en asilos de Tabasco y NL. *Animal Político*. Retrieved from https://www.animalpolitico.com/2020/05/brotes-covid-19-asilos-nl-tabasco/.

Redacción. (2020b, May 12). [Four older people die from Covid-19 in a Mexicali nursing home]. Fallecen cuatro adultos mayores por Covid-19 en asilo de Mexicali. *Aristegui Noticias*. Retrieved from https://aristeguinoticias.com/1205/mexico/fallecen-cuatro-adultos-mayores-por-covid-19-en-asilo-de-mexicali/.

Redacción. (2020c, May 17). [NL reports new outbreak of COVID-19 in nursing home and a baby with the coronavirus]. NL reporta nuevo brote de COVID-19 en asilo y a una bebé con el coronavirus. *Animal Político*. Retrieved from https://www.animalpolitico.com/2020/05/nl-nuevo-brote-asilo-covid-19-bebe/.

Redacción. (2020d, July 8). [COVID outbreak in Coahuila nursing home leaves two dead women and 15 infected]. Brote de COVID en asilo de Coahuila deja dos mujeres muertas y 15 contagiados. *Animal Político*. Retrieved from https://www.animalpolitico.com/2020/07/brote-covid-asilo-las-vinas-coahuila/.

Sakamoto, H., Rahman, M., Nomura, S., Okamoto, E., Yasunaga, H., Kawakami, N., Ghaznavi, C. (2018). Asia Pacific Observatory on Health Systems and Policies. In K. Shibuya, S. Gilmour, & K. Tatara (Eds.), *Japan Health System Review Health Systems in Transition* (Vol. 8). Retrieved from http://apps.who.int/iris/.

Salinas-Rodríguez, A., Torres-Pereda, M. D. P., Manrique-Espinoza, B., Moreno-Tamayo, K., & Téllez-Rojo Solís, M. M. (2014). Impact of the

Non-Contributory Social Pension Program 70 y más on Older people' Mental Well-Being. *PLoS ONE*, *9*(11), e113085. https://doi.org/10.1371/journal.pone.0113085.

Sanchéz, M., & Chio, Y. (2020, June 13). [Covid outbreak at home in Ciudad Victoria]. Brote de Covid en casa hogar de Ciudad Victoria. *La Jornada*. Retrieved from https://www.jornada.com.mx/2020/06/13/estados/026n2est.

Secretaria de Bienestar, P. (2020, June 26). [Sectorial Welfare PROGRAM 2020-2024]. PROGRAMA Sectorial de Bienestar 2020-2024. *Diario Oficial de La Federación*. Retrieved from http://www.dof.gob.mx/nota_detalle.php?codigo=5595663&fecha=26/06/2020.

Secretaria de Salud, P. (2019, September 27). [Project of Official Mexican Standard PROY-NOM-031-SSA3-2018, Social assistance. Provision of social assistance services to adults and older people in situations of risk and vulnerability.]. Proyecto de Norma Oficial Mexicana PROY-NOM-031-SSA3-2018, Asist. *Diario Oficial de La Federación*. Retrieved from http://www.dof.gob.mx/nota_detalle.php?codigo=5573764&fecha=27/09/2019.

Swartz, K. (2013). Searching for a balance of responsibilities: OECD countries' changing elderly assistance policies. *Annual Review of Public Health*, *34*, 397–412. https://doi.org/10.1146/annurev-publhealth-031912-114505.

The Green House Project. (2020). *The Green House Project Research Summary*. Retrieved October 13, 2020, from https://www.thegreenhouseproject.org/application/files/7215/9673/9561/GHP_Research_Summary_Nov_2019.pdf.

Tonantzin, P. (2020, July 30). [Covid-19 outbreak reported in Morelos nursing home]. *Reportan brote de Covid-19 en asilo de Morelos. Excelsior*. Retrieved from https://www.excelsior.com.mx/nacional/reportan-brote-de-covid-19-en-asilo-de-morelos/1381270.

United Nations Population Division. (n.d.). *UN data Life expectancy at birth for both sexes combined (years)*. Retrieved August 31, 2020, from https://data.un.org/Data.aspx?q=mexico&d=PopDiv&f=variableID%3A68%3BcrID%3A484.

Villalobos Dintrans, P. (2018). Long-term care systems as social security: The case of Chile. *Health Policy and Planning*, *33*(9), 1018–1025. https://doi.org/10.1093/heapol/czy083.

Wittenberg, R., & Malley, J. (2007). Financing Long-Term Care for Older People in England. *Ageing Horizons*, (6), 28-32. https://www.ageing.ox.ac.uk/download/37

World Health Organization. (2017). *Global strategy and action plan on ageing and health*. Retrieved from http://apps.who.int/bookorders.

World Health Organization. (2018). *WHO | Integrated Care for Older People.* Retrieved July 27, 2018, from WHO website: http://www.who.int/ageing/health-systems/icope/en/.

World Health Organization. (2019). *Integrated care for older people (ICOPE): Guidance for person-centred assessment and pathways in primary care.* Retrieved from https://apps.who.int/iris/bitstream/handle/10665/326843/WHO-FWC-ALC-19.1-eng.pdf?sequence=17.

World Health Organization. (2020). *Preventing and managing COVID-19 across long-term care services: Policy brief, 24 July 2020*. Retrieved from https://www.who.int/publications/i/item/WHO-2019-nCoV-Policy_Brief-Long-term_Care-2020.1.

Yourish, K., Rebeca, L. K. K., Ivory, D., & Smith, M. (2020). One-Third of All U.S. Coronavirus Deaths Are Nursing Home Residents or Workers. *The New York Times*. Retrieved from: https://www.nytimes.com/interactive/2020/05/09/us/coronavirus-cases-nursing-homes-us.html.

In: The Future of Long-Term Care
Editor: Pablo Villalobos Dintrans
ISBN: 978-1-53619-263-6

Chapter 7

THE LONG-TERM CARE INSURANCE SYSTEM IN SOUTH KOREA: OVERVIEW AND FUTURE CHALLENGES

Misook Song and Hyunjong Song*
[1]College of Nursing, Ajou University,
Suwon, Republic of Korea
[2]Department of Health Policy and Management,
College of Health Sciences, Sangji University,
Wonju, Republic of Korea

ABSTRACT

South Korea is experiencing rapid population aging with increased life expectancy and lowered fertility. The country has proactively launched long-term care services under a national social insurance system; services are paid for by a single insurer that has provided universal coverage since July 1st, 2008. The long-term care insurance (LTCI) program provides both in-home and institutional services, mainly targeting elderly who need assistance in daily living. As the LTCI system in South Korea has continued to extend its eligible population, service

* Corresponding Author's E-mail: igypop@hanmail.net.

coverage, and infrastructure for service provision, building a sustainable system has become an important policy agenda in the country. Therefore, South Korea's LTCI should strengthen measures to maintain financial sustainability, provide additional services to enable care in the home, create a mechanism to assure high care quality, and implement a coordination system to ensure continuity of care.

1. Aging and Social Change in South Korea

South Korea is an example of a rapidly aging country that is currently experiencing an accelerated process of demographic transition. According to the estimates of the Korean National Statistical Office, the ratio of people 65 years and older (65+) is expected to increase rapidly from 7.2% in 2000, to 20.3% in 2025, and 33.9% in 2040 (Statistics Korea, 2019). Figure 1 shows the aging trends in several countries. Compared to other countries, South Korea's aging process has been accelerating since 2000, and the proportion of people aged 65+ will be larger in the country than in Japan by 2060.

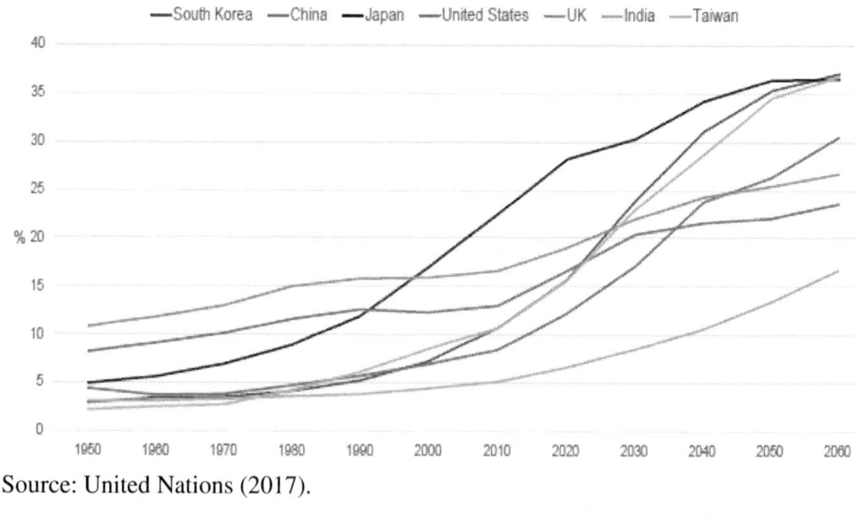

Source: United Nations (2017).

Figure 1. Percentage of people 65+ over of the total population in selected countries.

This trend resulted from a sharp decline in fertility rate and a rapid increase in life expectancy. In 2018, South Korea's total fertility rate was the lowest among OECD countries at 1.0 birth per woman (OECD, 2020), and this trend has continued for the past decade. By 2030, both Korean men and women are expected to have the longest life expectancy in the world (Kontis et al., 2017). The population structure of people 65+ is also expected to change. The Korean National Statistical Office reported that by 2067, the population aged 65 to 84 will start decreasing, while people aged 85 or older will exhibit a continuous increase. Accordingly, the population over 85 years will increase from 173,273 in 2000 to over 1 million in 2024, and to about 5 million by 2067. In relative terms, this increase implies that the share of people over 85 years will go from 1.2% of the total population in 2017 to 13.0% by 2067 (Korean National Statistical Office, 2019).

One of the main issues presented by the increase in the elderly population—especially in the oldest group—is the expected growth in the number of people needing care of some kind. According to a survey of living conditions of Korean older people (Table 1), which used a nationwide sample representative of community dwelling older people, 85.1% of those aged 65 or older had no functional restriction in 2011, but this decreased to 74.7% in 2017 (KIHASA, 2018). In addition, the restriction rate for instrumental activities of daily living (IADL) increased significantly in the same period, going from 7.7% to 16.6% (Table 1).

Table 1. Functional restriction rate among community dwelling elderly in South Korea (%)

Survey year	No restriction	IADL restriction	IADL + ADL restriction
2011	85.1	7.7	7.2
2014	81.8	11.3	6.9
2017	74.7	16.6	8.7

Source: KIHASA (2018).

Note: IADL: instrumental activities of daily living; ADL: basic activities of daily living.

Table 2. Number of dementia patients and prevalence in South Korea

Year	Number of patients	Prevalence (%)
2015	648,223	9.79
2020	840,010	10.39
2030	1,272,444	10.03
2040	1,964,056	11.90
2050	2,710,032	15.06
2060	2,950,231	16.74

Source: Kim et al., (2017).

Table 3. Attitudes toward living with children and place of residence in the future, 60 or older (%)

Year	Want to live with children		Desired place of residence when not wanting to live with children		
	Yes	No	Home	LTC Facility	Other
2009	37.1	62.9	77.1	20.8	2.1
2011	29.0	71.0	81.6	17.3	1.1
2013	27.0	73.0	78.8	20.6	0.7
2015	24.9	75.1	86.0	13.3	0.7
2017	22.2	77.8	87.4	12.6	0.0
2019	20.7	79.3	87.2	12.8	0.1

Source: Statistics Korea (2020).

On the other hand, persons with dementia present cognitive and behavioral disorders that interfere with their daily functioning and independent living. Global dementia prevalence has been estimated to increase at a fast pace, especially in low- and middle-income countries, where life expectancy is rising faster than high-income countries (Prince, 2015). South Korea's dementia prevalence is estimated to increase from 8.7% in 2010 to 15.1% in 2050, raising the number of dementia patients from about 420,000 in 2008 to about 2.71 million in 2050 (Kim et al., 2017). Because of this increase in dementia patients, social costs are expected to increase from 11.7 trillion won[1] in 2013 to 43.2 trillion won (1.5 percent of GDP) in 2050 (Kim et al., 2017).

[1] Approximately 1 US dollar = 1,100 Korean won.

Due to a decrease in the birth rate and an increase in the elderly population, the old age dependency ratio, which is the population aged 65+ divided by the population aged 15 to 64, will increase from 18.8 in 2017 to more than 50 in 2036. Furthermore, family structure and attitudes toward care for older people have changed during the last decade (Jeon & Kwon, 2017). In a similar vein, elderly people's expectancy about receiving care from their own children is changing with the times. A social survey carried out in the age group of people over 60 years showed that the proportion of respondents who want to live with their children was 37.1% in 2009, but in 2019, the rate decreased to 20.7%. This trend is expected to continue to decline in the future. On the other hand, in 2009, when asked about where they want to live, if not with their children, 20.8% of people over 60 years declared their preference to live in a facility, with 77.1% preferring to live at home. However, in 2019, the share of people who reported wanting to live in a facility had decreased (12.8%) and the proportion of respondents who want to stay at home had increased (87.2%). These results show that the number of older people who want to live independently in their own home without living with their children is increasing in South Korea.

2. Overview of Long-Term Care Insurance

The increase in the share of the population aged 65+ means a significant change in the country's long-term care (LTC) needs. In April 2007, the country passed Long-term Care Insurance (LTCI), the implementation of which started in July 2008, as the fifth social insurance in South Korea. The LTCI is a national social insurance that provides universal coverage.

As South Korea became an ageing society, the Korean government started to monitor the need for public, elderly LTC in 2000, with the launch of a Task Force Team (Won, 2013). In 2002, steering committees for the LTCI system—consisting of both scholars and public officers—was organized, and this team designed its framework and action plan for 2 years. And then, pilot operation of LTCI were conducted on several cities almost 3 years with preliminary draft of it. Finaly the LTCI was implemented in July 2008 after modifying the framework of LTCI based in the evaluation of pilot operation. The national LTCI is overseen by the Ministry of Health and Welfare (MOHW) and operated by the National Health Insurance Service (NHIS), the single public insurer. Figure 2 shows the governance structure of South Korean LTCI (Kim & Kwon, 2021).

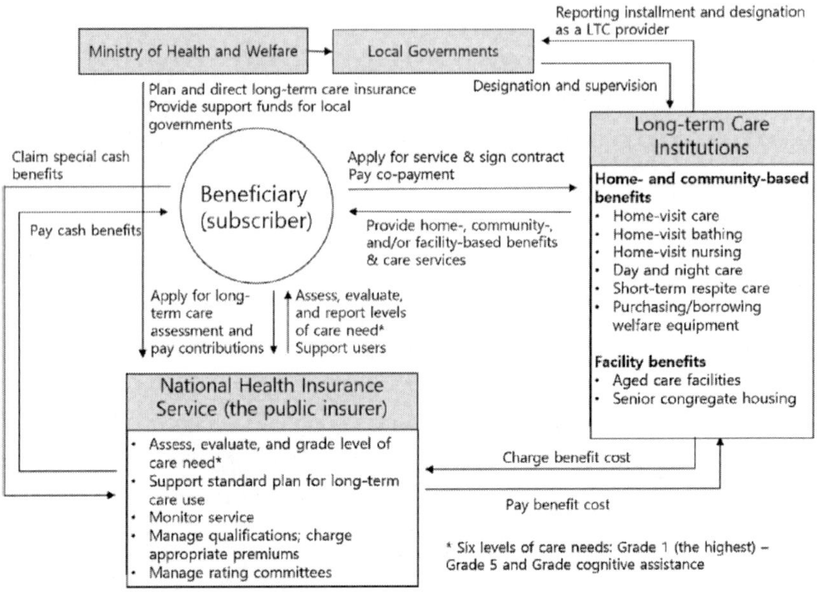

Source: Kim & Kwon (2021).

Figure 2. The management system of national LTCI in South Korea.

2.1. Eligibility for LTCI

Older people (aged 65 and over) can apply unconditionally for LTCI eligibility, but benefits for people under 65 are restricted to those that, due to age-related diseases (e.g., dementia, Parkinson's disease, or cerebrovascular disease), have limitations in performing daily life activities (Kim & Kwon, 2021). The process starts with the person (or person's caregiver) submitting an application form, along with a doctor's medical opinion, to the NHIS. NHIS staff members visit the applicant's house to examine his/her condition and approve the application for the system's benefits, using a checklist for LTC needs. The LTC needs assessment checklist, which consisted of 52 items, evaluates the presence of diseases, physical functioning, cognitive functioning, behavioral changes, nursing needs (Table 4).

Table 4. The 52-item checklist for assessing LTC needs

Domain	Item	Response option
Activities of daily living (12)	Dressing, washing face, brushing teeth, bathing, eating, turning in bed, sitting up in bed, transfer from bed to chair, moving out of room, toileting, bowel control, bladder control	Independent/ Partially dependent/ Fully dependent
Cognitive function (7)	Short-term memory, remembering dates, places, date of birth, understanding instructions, judgment, communication	Yes/No
Problem behaviors (14)	Feeling persecuted, visual or auditory hallucination, depressed mood, reversal of day and night, resisting advice or care, restlessness, being lost, verbal or physical violence, trying to go out alone, destroying items, meaningless behavior, hiding money or items, dressing inappropriately, unsanitary behavior	Yes/No
Nursing care needs (9)	Tracheostomy care, suction, oxygen therapy, sore care, tube feeding, pain control, urine catheter care, colostomy care, dialysis care	Yes/No
Rehabilitation needs (10)	Motor disturbance in right arm, left arm, right leg, left leg; limitation of movement in joints in shoulder, elbow, wrist, hip, knee, ankle	Not disabled/ Partially disabled/ Disabled No limitation/ Limitation of one joint/ Limitation of both joints

Source: Won (2013).

The results of the assessment are used to estimate the care time needed for each applicant, which is standardized on the basis of 100 points in a scale called the Long-term Care Approval Score. This system was developed by applying a decision-tree model, using the health and functional status information in the LTC needs assessment checklist. The LTC Need Assessment Committee rates applicants according to the time required for LTC by referring to the checklist results, which specify the applicant's mental and physical condition, along with a medical opinion. LTCI applicants are categorized into seven groups (Grade 1~5, Grade Cognition Assistance, Outside Grades) based on the severity of the beneficiary's care needs. Grade 1 includes those with the highest level of care needs, while those in Grade 5 have the lowest care needs. Grade Cognition Assistance is assigned to the applicants with mild dementia but with relatively good physical functioning. Among these groups, applicants of Grade 1 to 5 and Grade Cognition Assistance are serviced by LTCI, and community caring services not covered by LTCI are available for applicants who are assigned to Outside Grades. The current rating system has been applied since 2018.

Once an applicant is approved for an LTC grade, the NHIS issues a Standard Care Plan, which is written by NHIS care personnel (who are not required by the NHIS to have any license or certification). The Standard Care Plan recommends the type and quantity of services that can be used within the monthly limit derived by the computerized algorithm called the Standard Benefit Model. This plan includes information about service types, frequency of each service type, benefit costs, and out-of-pocket costs recommended by the NHIS. In South Korean LTCI, although there is no official care management service, the Standard Care Plan acts as a basis for making the service contract between providers and beneficiaries.

2.2. Types of Benefits

South Korea's LTCI benefits are classified into in-home services (home-visit caring, home-visit bathing, home-visit nursing, day-and-night care, short-term respite care, and medical-equipment rental), institutional services, and special cash benefits. Helping with ADLs, emotional support, and housekeeping are included in the home-visit caring benefits. Special cash benefits are recommended to only a small number of beneficiaries living in regions with a shortage of available LTC service institutions. By law, LTCI benefits are differentially recommended to beneficiaries based on their Grade (Table 5).

Table 5. Grading and recommended benefits of LTCI

Grade	Status	Recommended benefits
Grade 1	Completely dependent in activity of daily living	In-home services, Institutional services
Grade 2	Mostly dependent in activity of daily living	
Grade 3	Partially dependent in activity of daily living	In-home services
Grade 4	Mental and physical disabilities and partially dependent in activity of daily living	
Grade 5	Dementia and independent in activity of daily living	Day-and-night care, Home-visit care
Grade Cognitive Assistant		Day-and-night care, Short-term respite care

Source: NHIS (2020).

In principle, in-home care benefits should be provided to all LTCI beneficiaries by law. Grade 1 and 2 can use both in-home services and institutional services, but Grade 3~5 can use only in-home services except in exceptional cases (e.g., poor home environment, serious behavioral problem, and insufficient family care). Beneficiaries who are in Grade Cognitive Assistant can utilize only day-and-night care among in-home services. Institutional services are provided in small groups homes (≤9 persons) and nursing homes (≥10 persons) divided by institutionalized persons.

South Korea's LTCI includes specialized benefits for dementia beneficiaries through the Korean National Dementia Plans implemented by MOHW. A cognitive training program based on home visiting or specialized dementia care in nursing homes is provided to dementia beneficiaries.

2.3. The Standards of Staffing for LTC Facilities

Long term care staffs include RNs (Registered Nurse) or CNAs (Certified Nursing Assistant), certified care workers, social workers, and physical or occupational therapists. Most of custodial care and housekeeping assistance for beneficiaries who have limitation in ADL is performed by care worker mainly. They are qualified with certification which is issued by the Ministry of Health and Welfare (MOHW) after completing 240 hours of education and taking a qualification test. However, additional training is required to take care of beneficiaries with dementia in order to provide cognitive training programs. Care worker who wants to take care of resident with dementia should receive additional training to provide cognitive enhancement programs for them.

RN is responsible for the whole process of caring, such as assessment of care needs, supervision of the CAN, wound care, management of medication and pain control, etc. in nursing home. By the way, the scope of practice for CAN in a Korean nursing home is similar to that of a Licensed Practice Nurse (LPN) in the United States (Song & Song, 2019). For being a CAN, educational requirements are 740 hours of classroom study at an occupational high school or a private nursing academy and over 780 hours of clinical practice.

The MOHW sets the standard of staffing for each type of LTC facilities as follows: For nursing home, one RN or CAN to 25 residents, and one care worker to 2.5 residents are required by legal minimum standard. In nursing home that has more than 29 beds, there is at least one physical or occupational therapist. This standard also requires at least one social worker who is responsible for designing care plans for residents and consulting for resident's family. RN or CAN, certified care workers, and physical or occupation therapist directly provide services to residents in institutional care facility not in group home according to minimum staffing standards. Because for group homes, a lower minimum-staffing standard than for nursing home is applied, one care worker to 3 residents, and one RN or CAN or physical or occupational therapist are required.

2.4. Financing and Reimbursement

Contribution-based social insurance financing was adopted at the time of launching LTCI in South Korea. The South Korean welfare state is based on various social insurance schemes such as health insurance, pensions, unemployment insurance, and workplace injury compensation.

By making use of the existing administrative structure of the health insurer, the National Health Insurance Corporation (NHIC), LTCI minimized administrative costs (Kwon, 2009).

A major source of financing is the contributions that are collected from all participants of the National Health Insurance system. Besides individual contributions, there are three additional sources of financing (Rhee et al., 2015). First, the government supplements the LCTI contributions with additional funding from general taxes, which represents 20% of the anticipated contribution receipts by the LTCI law. Second, state and local governments subsidize the full contribution for those eligible for welfare benefits (called the Basic Livelihood Security Program, BLSP). They subsidize 50% of the contribution for the second-poorest group of citizens, who most often live in poverty but do not meet the strict eligibility requirements for the BSLP, which includes income, assets, and the availability of assistance by relatives. Finally, copayments are set at 15% of costs for in-home services and 20% for institutional care services. Even though the poor are exempted from these copayments, high out-of-pocket expenses have raised concerns about unaffordability of services, especially for the near poor (Rhee et al., 2015). In the case of institutional care, costs for food, haircuts and hairstyling, upgraded rooms, and other services are not covered by LTCI.

Payment schemes vary by benefit type. Institutional care (including group homes) and short-term respite care are reimbursed on a pay-per-day basis. Home-visit caring, home-visit nursing, and day-and-night care are reimbursed on a pay-per-hour basis, and home-visit bathing are reimbursed on a pay-per-visit basis (Kim & Kwon, 2021). LTC personnel providing services pertaining to additional staff (e.g., social workers, nursing personnel) over the minimum staff standard are reimbursed at extra cost. There are ceilings on the monthly benefits for in-home services. In 2020, the ceiling ranged from 1,007,200 to 1,498,300 Korean won (approximately from 916 US dollar to 1,362 US dollar), depending on the LTC grade. For Grade Cognitive Assistant, the maximum cost ceiling is 566,500 Korean won (approximately 515 US dollar) (MOHW, 2019). The fee schedule, including the ceiling for benefits, is reviewed and modified annually by LTC committee based on the LTCI Act.

3. Development and Future Policy Challenges for Long-term Care Insurance

3.1. Population Coverage and Financial Sustainability

Since the introduction of LTCI, the number of people who were enrolled for LTCI has increased significantly due to increased public awareness of the related policy. The introduction of a policy to expand targets was critical to increasing participation of the elderly with deteriorating functions. From 2008 to 2011, the number of targets increased rapidly due to the increase in public awareness of the system, and the increase of targets from 2012 to 2015 can be seen as the effect of the annual policy to lower the approval score.

Table 6. Population coverage under the national LTIC in South Korea

		2008	2009	2012	2014	2016	2018	2019
Population aged 65+ (number)		5,086,195	5,286,383	5,921,977	6,462,740	6,940,396	7,611,770	8,003,418
Applicants (number)		355,526	522,293	643,409	736,879	848,829	1,009,209	1,113,093
Total certified (number)		214,480	286,907	341,788	424,572	519,850	670,810	772,206
Proportion of grade (%)	Grade 1	26.8	16.8	11.2	8.9	7.9	6.7	5.8
	Grade 2	27.2	25.4	20.7	17.0	14.3	12.6	11.2
	Grade 3	46.0	57.9	68.1	40.1	35.7	31.5	29.3
	Grade 4				31.6	36.3	39.5	42.2
	Grade 5				2.5	5.8	8.0	9.5
	Grade Cognition Assistance						1.7	2.0
Certified compared to population aged 65+ (%)		4.2	5.4	5.8	6.6	7.5	8.8	9.6
LTC benefit recipients (number)		149,656	291,389	369,587	433,779	520,043	648,792	732,181

Source: NHIS (2020).

From 2012 to 2014, the number of approval scores was lowered by 4 points, and about 82,000 eligible persons were in flow during this period. Since the establishment of LTCI, the number of certified people increased by about 2.7 times, from 287,907 in 2009 (5.4% of the 65 years or older elderly) to 772,206 in 2019 (9.6% of the 65 years or older elderly). The LTCI was implemented in July 2008, so the statistics for 2008 are only for half the year. The proportion of Grade 3 and below increased rather than the proportion of severe beneficiaries of Grade 1 and 2. This is a result of LTCI target expansion policy that has newly incorporated the elderly with relatively mild care needs (Table 6). As the prevalence of dementia increases, the share of elderly dementia patient among LTC certified people is also increasing.

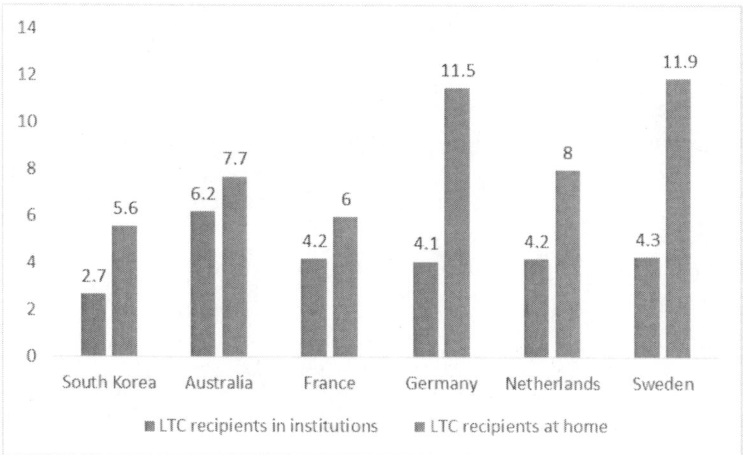

Source: OECD (2020).

Figure 3. Proportion of LTC recipients of total population aged 65+ by type of benefits in South Korea among some OECD countries, 2017.

Table 7. LTCI expenditure in South Korea (billion, Korean won)

	2009	2012	2014	2016	2018	2019
Total LTCI revenue	2,085	3,562	4,149	4,730	6,153	7,620
Total LTCI expenditure	1,908	2,937	3,850	4,723	6,801	8,315
Balance	177	625	299	7	-648	-695

Source: NHIS (2020).

Figure 3 shows the coverage rates of LTCI in South Korea compared to OECD countries. This data was calculated as the number of LTC recipients among the population aged 65+. The coverage rate in Korea is still low compared to that of major OECD countries, especially with respect to in-home service. Accordingly, one of the policy tasks of LCTI in Korea is to expand the number of eligible people (Lee et al., 2018). However, these policies should be pursued while also considering financial stability.

The current account balance for 2018 and 2019 was in the red, as LTCI spending increased annually. However, as MOHW is planning a policy to increase the number of LTCI beneficiaries, the utilization of LTCI is expected to increase, so there are concerns about financial stability. As about 65% of Korea's LTCI financing sources depend on individual contributions, it is necessary to discuss the diversification of this financing. In unexpected situations such as COVID-19 in 2020, financial sustainability can be threatened if the proportion of dependence on individual contributions is high.

3.2. Need-Based Services for "Aging in Place" and People's Preferences

In 2018, Korea's Ministry of Health and Welfare announced the implementation of the "Community Care" policy, which enables people in need of care to utilize welfare services that meet their needs while living with others in community (Lee, 2018). Older adults were set as the first target of the policy in consideration of the rate of aging in Korean society. To implement this policy, the government announced a plan to develop a measure to merge health and social care. Increasing in-home service utilization by expanding the quantity and improving the quality of in-home services was proposed as one of the specific ways to accomplish policy implementation.

The South Korean "Community Care" policy serves the symbolic and philosophical concept of "Aging in Place." "Aging in Place" is a popular term in current aging policy (Wiles et al., 2011), defined as "having people remain in their homes and community for as long as possible maintaining independence, autonomy by providing social and health support." As mentioned earlier in this chapter, the number of elderly people who prefer independent living at home is increasing, which implies that specific measures to realize "Aging in Place" within the LTCI of Korea should be included. In other words, LTCI services should match the need of LTCI beneficiaries.

Many European countries employ care management to promote in-home care-centered community care that combines health and social care (Leichsening, 2004) for meeting elderly's "Aging in Place" needs. The Korean LTC insurer issues a Standard Care Plan that contains the goals of LTC and amount of needed services legislated by LTCI Act (Song & Song, 2020), similar to the care plans in other countries. In addition, the policy direction for pursuing "Aging in Place" is stated in the LTCI Act, that in-home service benefits should be provided first to LTC beneficiary. Despite these efforts, concerns are raised frequently that in-home services covered by Korea's LTCI are inappropriate in quantity, type, and quality relative to the needs of beneficiaries (Chon, 2018).

First, in-home services such as home-visit caring, home-visit bathing, home-visit nursing, day-and-night care, short-term respite care, and medical-equipment rental are provided separately under a different fee schedule for each benefit, and beneficiaries must choose the services below the coverage ceiling. Furthermore, in making the Standard Care Plan, only specific needs are reflected. Therefore, home-visit caring was recommended to over 85% of LTC beneficiaries regardless of LTC Grade (Song & Song, 2015). Due to the maximum monthly allowance in using in-home care benefits, LTC beneficiaries tend to choose inexpensive home-visit caring instead of expensive home-visit nursing. Home-visit caring accounts for around 70% of the LTCI expenditures for in-home services, while home-visit nursing comprises less than 1%.

There were 8,446 home-visit caring institutions in 2009, a number which almost doubled in 2019. However, during the same period, the number of home-visit nursing institutions increased from 787 to 795.

Table 8. Share of LTCI expenditures by in-home benefit type (%)

In-home benefit type	2008	2009	2012	2014	2016	2019
Home-visit caring	66.2	74.4	82.2	78.3	73.8	68.8
Home-visit bathing	5.8	4.1	5.0	4.2	3.5	2.7
Home-visit nursing	0.9	0.6	0.4	0.5	0.4	0.5
Day-and-night care	10.7	6.3	5.3	10.4	16.6	23.9
Short-term respite care	9.4	8.6	2.3	1.0	0.6	0.3
Medical equipment rental	7.1	6.0	4.6	5.6	5.2	3.9

Source: NHIS (2020).

Table 9. Number of in-home service institutions

In-home benefit type	2008	2009	2012	2014	2016	2019
Home-visit caring	4,206	8,446	8,500	9,073	11,072	15,305
Home-visit bathing	2,959	6,279	7,028	7,479	8,957	11,121
Home-visit nursing	592	787	626	586	598	795
Day-and-night care	790	1,106	1,331	1,688	2,410	4,179
Short-term respite care	694	1,368	257	322	267	162
Medical equipment rental	720	1,086	1,498	1,599	1,823	1,975

Source: NHIS (2020).

A previous study (Yoo et al., 2016) reported that although LTC beneficiaries typically have 2 or 3 chronic diseases, 84.3% of them use only home-visiting caring services or a mix of home-visiting caring and home-visit bathing. Song & Song (2020) reported that disagreement between insurer-recommended home care services and beneficiary-selected institution services increased with age, having high care needs, dementia, and poor subjective hearing. Under these circumstances, LTCI beneficiaries whose medical problem and symptoms have worsened are forced to use hospitals. To prevent beneficiaries suffering from medical problems from being admitted to facilities by management of home-visiting nurses, the LTCI system needs to be improved. To overcome this limitation, NHIS has conducted pilot projects, called integrated home services, since 2016. A previous study (Yoo et al, 2020) reported that although positive overall results have been achieved in providing customized services to target beneficiaries through the use of integrated home-services, it has been difficult to change the existing service supply pattern and has limitations with regard to providing an effective linkage between care and medical services.

Second, several studies showed that the Standard Care Plan has deficiencies in reflecting LTC needs and preferences of the beneficiary and family (Song & Song, 2018) and has relatively low compliance (Lee et al., 2008; Song & Song, 2020). Establishing the validity of the Standard Care Plan, which acts as care management for Korean LTCI, and having beneficiaries adhere to it are crucial for executing "Aging in Place" policy. First, NHIS prepares the Standard Care Plan without considering the values and preferences of caregivers or beneficiaries. Since caregiver preference is a major factor affecting LTC service choice (Shyu & Lee, 2002; Choi & Joung, 2016), it must be considered in care management. Because care plans in Korea are prepared by the insurer, problems about provider-induced demands for care services, as in the case of Japan, are rarely called into question (Campbell & Ikegami, 2000). However, in Japan, the community care center assesses the appropriateness of benefit usage and satisfaction and frequently communicates with the elderly person and caregiver for the selection of a care-providing institution during the process of preparing the care plan. For supporting aging in place, the concession of greater flexibility in packaging care services should be developed to increase autonomy and caring capacity of families with dependent members (Pavolini & Ranci, 2008). However, the Standard Care Plan is issued annually following the LTCI care needs assessment, which could fail to promptly respond to the changing physical and mental status and the care environment of beneficiaries. In addition, there is no assessment of adherence after issuing the Standard Care Plan. To promote appropriate use of care benefits, it is important to assess the physical and emotional care environment at home to maintain the continuity of service between family members or caregivers and the LTC service provider. However, under the current system, the insurer does not make any assessments regarding this matter. In order to achieve the purpose of the care plan, it is recommended that it be prepared based on the understanding of the integrated needs assessment through active intervention by medical personnel, more actively reflect the preferences and opinions of the recipients and their families, and be modified whenever the beneficiary's care needs change.

Third, in addition to reflecting the needs of family caregivers when issuing the Standard Care Plan, practical support for them is needed. In Korean LTCI, two types of family caregiving (special cash benefit and family caregiver certified by MOHW) are officially recognized. Special cash benefits are provided to beneficiaries who are living in regions with a shortage of available LTC service institutions and are cared for by family caregivers. If family caregivers who have obtained a certification issued by MOHW provide home-visit caring, NHIS pays them as LTC providers. Although Korea established the LTCI system, family caregiving is provided due to elderly person's desire to be protected by their family. Despite NHIS reducing the scope of benefits by family care workers, it was found that the number of recipients receiving benefits from family workers has been increased from 37,000 in 2010 to 42,000 in 2016 (Lee, 2018). Previous studies (Han et al., 2015; Song & Song, 2020) reported that the burden on family caregivers was considerable, especially dementia beneficiaries' family caregivers. Therefore, a supportive care environment should be provided for families to provide care for beneficiaries, and insurance benefits should be modified to ensure their continuity of care. Also, respite and counseling services are necessary to relieve the burden on family caregivers.

3.3. Quality Assurance System

In the early stage of LTCI launching, there was a consensus that the LTCI could not be implemented without an adequate supply of providers, so the Government allocated funds for building LTC institutions and renovating existing facilities, as well as the promotion of private sector participation (Rhee et al., 2015). As the number of LTC institutions increased, quality of care became a crucial issue due to the broad spectrum of quality across LTC institutions (Kwon, 2009).

In Korean LTCI, there are two major policy measures for ensuring quality of care: one is financial incentive based on quality evaluation, and the other is accreditation and renewal. While NHIS conducts the entire process of evaluating quality of care, local governments are responsible for accreditation of LTC providers. A quality evaluation system for LTC facilities has been implemented at a national level, based on current law. The first nationwide quality inspection was conducted in 2009 on a voluntary basis, and the inspection was mandated in 2010, with repetition every 3 years (Kim & Kwon, 2021). The quality evaluation for nursing homes started in 2009 and extended to all kinds of LTC facilities in 2011.

In evaluating the quality of LTC facilities, frameworks of structures, processes, and outcomes (SPO) proposed by Donabedian are widely used (Castle & Ferguson, 2010), but recently, composite measures including the mixture of structures, processes, and outcomes have emerged. The Nursing Home Compare operated by CMS (Center for Medicare & Medicaid Services) is one example, which includes a comprehensive scope of quality indicators at a national scale. Korea also classifies nursing homes into five grades (A-E grade) based on the composite evaluation indicators (Song & Song, 2019). Indicators about operational management, environment and safety, residents' rights, service processes, and outcomes are used for evaluating. Financial incentives are paid by adding a certain percentage to the reimbursement size of a LTC facility. The additional percentage is determined by the budget range allocated to the incentive item for this year. Furthermore, the Korean government instituted a mandatory regulatory public-reporting system (Shin et al., 2020) for ensuring the public's right to know and increasing the public's knowledge when choosing an LTC service provider. Results of the evaluation are released to the public through the NHIS website.

Accreditation is the process by which a (non-)governmental or private body evaluates the quality of an institution as a whole or of a specific program in order to formally recognize it as having met certain pre-determined minimum criteria or standards (Vlasceanu et al., 207). It is usually a voluntary program, in which trained external peer reviewers evaluate (Shaw, 2004). In Korea, all organizations that intend to be designated as LTC providers should apply for accreditation with a document that contains information about staff, the facility, and plans for services to local government. Local government examines the application on the basis of the mandatory standards concerning staff, facilities, etc. The duration of validity of the accreditation is 6 years, and LTC providers are able to renew their accreditation according to the decision of local government.

Although the LTC quality evaluation system that is composed of regular quality evaluations and accreditations was initiated to improve the quality of care, there are still several limitations with this system. First, since accreditation is based on compliance with minimum legal standards, these standards are critical in determining quality of care in LTCI. Especially, standards about staffing affect the quality of care because LTCI services require a large number of human services, rather than medical services (Song & Song, 2019). In Korean LTCI, since the fee schedule for LTC providers is set under a prepayment system according to minimum staffing standards, this affects financial aspects of facilities. A previous study (Lee et al., 2015) reported that Korea has lower registered nurse and certified nursing assistant standards and actual staffing levels than the United States. In contrast, staffing standards for care workers who provide direct care to residents are higher in Korea than the United States and Japan (Chin & Lee, 2012). Furthermore, because nursing staff, regardless of whether RN or can, is included in the minimum mandatory personnel in Korean LTCI, detailed monitoring for change in LTC beneficiary clinical status is limited. A previous study (Korean Health Insurance Policy Institute, 2012) proposed a new staffing standard in nursing homes that included a ratio of one RN or CNA per 20 residents (instead of per 25 residents), the mandated use of an advanced practice nurse, and one RN for every two CNAs. The proposal was not accepted for several reasons, primarily financial burden.

Second, the reliability and validity of quality assurance system in LTCI is being raised continuously. Since most of the evaluation indicators are assessed based on the documentation drawn up by LTC provider, it does not evaluate the actual service provision process and outcomes. Due to insufficient number of outcome-based indicators, a gap between real quality of care and evaluation results exists. Currently, the NHIS evaluates prevalence of pressure ulcers and urinary tract infections, function of controlling bowels or bladder, and changes in LTC grade as outcome indicators for nursing homes.

Considering that CMS applies 23 quality measures (QM) for long stay residents in nursing homes based on the MDS (Minimum Data Set) using RAI (Resident Assessment Instrument) (CMS, 2020), the number of outcome indicators using by the NHIS evaluation is relatively few. Since the evaluation period mandated in LTCI law is 3 years, it is not possible to examine the changes in LTC service provision and outcomes between evaluations. Therefore, improvement of quality evaluation indicators and methods are required on the on-site inspection, including standardized, resident-level indicators for assessing quality of care, health outcomes, and quality of life (Kim et al., 2015).

Finally, for ensuring adequate LTC providers quality nationwide, interventions targeted to low-quality institutions are necessary. Although NHIS reported that the quality of LTC institutions is improving over time, low-quality providers still exist. It is required more active intervention by NHIS rather than waiting for these institutions to improve the quality of their services themselves. A whip strategy for institutions providing inappropriate services and a carrot strategy for superior institutions are needed at the same time (Lee, 2011).

CONCLUSION

South Korea introduced national LTCI to reduce the burden of excessive costs of LTC on individuals and their families in July 2008. South Korea's LTCI had the effect of lowering the social burden of elderly care by expanding the targets and service providers within a short period of time after its introduction. However, in order to expand the supply of services at the beginning of the system, there are limitations of demand versus supply control and quality assurance. In addition, because customized beneficiary management, such as the establishment and monitoring of the Standard Care Plan, was insufficient, individualized services according to the care needs and preferences of each elderly person were inadequate. Policy to expand the target population is continuously implemented in response to the increasing demand for care, which threatens the financial sustainability of LTCI. Under these circumstances, there are several key policy issues to be addressed in order to make South Korea's LTCI more person-centered and sustainable.

First, considering the increase in the aging population, the coverage rate of LTCI in Korea should be expanded. However, it is necessary to set an appropriate scale and establish a long-term plan. To do this, social consensus on who needs LTCI services is required, and the current LTCI eligibility evaluation system needs to be reorganized based on consensus.

Second, the Korean LTCI system does not seem to take into account the concept of person-centered care, this is because NHIS does not reflect a beneficiaries' care environment or their preference for LTC service at all when making the Standard Care Plan. Moreover it cannot be provided under such an insufficient mandatory standard of staffing in LTC facility. Therefore, it is necessary to upgrade the current labor force standard to level that can provide person-centered care. Reinforcement of nursing staff beyond the range of legal staffing that is currently stipulated is indispensable, and for this, a reorganization of the payment system must also occur. In addition, a systematic on-the-job training program for workers should be established, and an active disincentive policy should be introduced for low quality institutions. Recently, a pilot project for integration of segmented in-home benefits is being implemented, but there are difficulties with this that are mainly due to limitations in the payment system. For person-centered care in LTCI, caring for the beneficiary of dementia should be considered. With the rapid aging of Korea's population, services for the elderly and their families with dementia should be strengthened. Currently, the system is still insufficient to provide services suitable for the needs of the elderly with dementia, so many in this population use hospitals instead of LTCI services.

Third, it is necessary to guarantee the continuum of care by linkage of community-based and LTCI services. Applicants who do not get LTCI eligibility can receive community services and services for preventing LTC needs that are included in LTCI. LTC prevention services have not yet been provided, but they are necessary to manage the elderly that will have LTCI needs. This requires cooperation between the local government and the NHIS.

Finally, there is an issue in terms of LTCI governance. Governance is a function of the state, yet it cannot function without all actors across the LTC system, which includes civil societies, private providers, and membership organizations (Siddiqi et al., 2009). In Korea's LTCI, the local government and NHIS are in charge of operating LTCI, but cooperation between the two parties is insufficient. In addition, there is a lack of channels for the elderly and their families to express opinions related to the operation of LTCI. Therefore, it is necessary to prepare a plan to establish integrated governance between the NHIS and local governments, and to enable active participation of the elderly and their families.

REFERENCES

Campbell, J. C. and Ikegami, N. (2000). Long-Term Care Insurance comes to Japan. *Health Affairs*, 19 (3), 26-39.

Castle, N. G. and Ferguson, J. C. (2010). What is nursing home quality and how is it measured? *The Gerontologist*, 50 (4), 426-442.

Chin, Y. and Lee, H. Y. (2012). Comparing standards and guidelines of long-term care facilities based on physical environment and manpower in Korea, Japan, USA, and Australia. *Korean Journal of Health Policy & Administration*, 22 (3), 403-426.

Choi, J. and Joung, E. (2016). The association between the utilization of long-term care services and mortality in elderly Koreans. *Archives of Gerontology & Geriatrics*, 65, 122-127.

Chon Y. (2018). The use and coordination of the medical, public health and social care services for the elderly in terms of continuum of care. *Health and Social Welfare Review*, 38(4), 10-39.

CMS. (2020). *MDS 3.0 Quality Measures user's manual.*

Han, E. J., Na, Y., Lee, J. S., and Kwon, J. (2015). Factors to influence the family caregiver's burden with the community-dwelling elderly under long-term care insurance system: Comparison among sub-dimensions. *Korea Social Policy Review*, 6, 61-96.

Jeon, B. and Kwon, S. (2017). Health and long-term care systems for older people in the Republic of Korea: Policy challenges and lessons. *Health Systems & Reform*, 3 (3), 214-223.

KIHASA. (2018). *Survey of living conditions of Korean older people.* Sejong: KIHASA.

Kim, H. and Kwon, S. (2021). A decade of public long-term care insurance in South Korea: Policy lessons for aging countries. *Health Policy*, 125 (1), 22-26.

Kim, H., Jung, Y. I., and Kwon, S. (2015). Delivery of institutional long-term care under two social insurances: lessons from the Korean experience. *Health Policy*, 119, 1330-1337.

Kim, K. W., Kwak, K. P., Kim, B. S., Kim, B. J., Kim, J. R., Kim, T. H., Moon, S. W., Park, K. W., Park, J. I., Park, J. H., Seo, J. Y., Sung, S. J., Son, S. J., Sin, I. S., Yoo, S. H., Lee, K. J., Lee, S. B., Lee, J. J., Jung, H. K., Cho, S. J., Choi, Y. M., Han, J. W., Kim, K. W., Nam, H. J., and Ahn, J. Y. (2017). *Nationwide survey on the dementia epidemiology of Korea*. Seoul: MOHW.

Kontis, V., Bennett, J. E., Mathers, C. D., Li, G., Foreman, K. and Ezzati, M. (2017). Future life expectancy in 35 industrialised countries: projections with a Bayesian model ensemble. *The Lancet*, 389(10076), P1323-1335.

Korean Health Insurance Policy Institute. (2012). *Policy proposals about health care needs of long term care residents*. Seoul: NHIS.

Kwon, S. (2009). The introduction of long-term care insurance in South Korea. *Eusohealth* 15 (1), 28-29.

Lee, H. Y., Shin, J. H. and Harrington, C. (2015). Comparing the nurse staffing in Korea and U.S. nursing homes. *Nursing Outlook*, 63: 137-143.

Lee, K. (2018). Health care perspective on community care. *Journal of Korean Medical Association*, 61 (1), 586-589.

Lee, Y. K. (2011). Review of long-term care institution evaluation system and policy tasks. *Issue & Focus*, 92: 1-8.

Lee, Y. K. (2018). Current status of and barriers to home and community care in the Long-term Care System. *Health and Welfare Forum,* 5, 77-89.

Lee, Y. K., Jung, H., Seok, J. E., Song, H., Seo, D. M., Lee, J. S., Yoo, A. J., Lee, H. Y., Kwon, J. H., Kim, C., Park, J., Um, K., Lee, M. H., Jang, S., Chon, Y., Jung, J., Sunwoo, D., Kang, E., Sin, W., Lee, S., and Bae, H. (2018). *The 2nd Long-term Care Plan*. Sejong: KIHASA.

Leichsenring, K. (2004). Developing integrated health and social care services for older persons in Europe. *International Journal of Integrated Care*, 4 (3), 1-15.

NHIS. (2020). *Long Term Care Insurance statistical Yearbook*. Wonju: NHIS.

Pavolini, E. and Ranci, C. (2008). Restructuring the welfare state: Reforms in long-term care in Western European countries. *Journal of European Social Policy*, 18 (3), 246-259.

Prince, M., Wilmo, A., Guerchet, M., Ali, G., Wu, Y., and Prina, M. (2015). *World Alzheimer Report 2015: The global impact of dementia*. London: ADI.

Rhee, J. C. Done, N., and Anderson, G. F. (2015). Considering long-term care insurance for middle-income countries: comparing South Korea with Japan and Germany. *Health Policy,* 119, 1319-1329.

Shaw, C. D. (2004). *Toolkit for accreditation programs*. Australia: The International Society for Quality in Health Care.

Shin, J. H., Shin, I., and Lee, J. Y. (2020). Factors influencing nursing home accreditation-quality ratings in Korea. *Journal of Korean Gerontological Nursing*, 22 (3), 226-235.

Shyu, Y. L and Lee, H. (2002). Predictors of nursing home placement and home nursing services utilization by elderly patients after hospital discharge in Taiwan. *Journal of Advanced Nursing*, 38 (4): 398-406.

Siddiqi, S., Masud, T. I., Nishtar, S., Peters, D. H., Sabri, B., Bile, K. M., and Jama, M. A. (2009). Framework for assessing governance of the health system in developing countries: Gateway to good governance. *Health Policy*, 90 (1), 13-25.

Song, M. and Song, H. (2015). A study of the factors associated with home-based benefit recommendation of the Standard Utilization Plan in Long-term Care Insurance: Focusing on adequacy of Standard Utilization Plan. *Korean Journal of Gerontological Social Welfare*, 69, 31-49.

Song, M. and Song, H. (2018). Factors affecting 3~5grade beneficiaries' preference for utilization of facility care in Long-term Care Insurance. *Korean Journal of Gerontological Social Welfare*, 73 (4), 281-301.

Song, M. and Song, H. (2019). Staff mix and nursing home quality by level of case mix in Korea. *Geriatrics & Gerontology International*, 19, 438-443.

Song, M. and Song, H. (2020). Disagreement between a public insurer's recommendation and beneficiary's choice of long-term care service in Korea. *Health Policy*, 124, 881-887.

Statistics Korea. (2019). *Population statistics*. Daejeon: Statistics Korea.

Statistics Korea. (2020). *Social survey*. Daejeon: Statistics Korea.

United Nations. (2017). *World population prospects*.

Vlasceanu, L., Grunberg, L., and Parlea, D. (2007). *Quality assurance and accreditation: A glossary of basic terms and definitions*. UNESCO.

Wiles, J. L., Leibing, A., Guberman, N., Reeve, J., and Allen, R. E. S. (2011). The meaning of "Aging in Place" to older people. *The Gerontologist*, 52 (3), 357-366.

Won, C. W. (2013). Elderly long-term care in Korea. *Journal of Clinical Gerontology & Geriatrics*, 4, 4-6.

Yoo, A. J., Lee, J. S., and Park, S. Y. (2020). A study on the experience of long-term care facility operators to participate in the 3rd pilot project of integrated home-service. *Korean Journal of Gerontological Social Welfare*, 75 (2), 283-304.

Yoo, A. J., Lee, J. S., Han, E., and Na, Y. K. (2016). *Evaluation of 1st pilot project of integraed home-service in Long-term Care Insurance*. Seoul: NHIS.

About the Editor

Pablo Villalobos Dintrans is Commercial Engineer with a major in Economics and Master in Economics (concentration in public policy) from the Pontificia Universidad Católica de Chile. He also holds a Master of Arts in economics from Boston University and a Doctorate in Public Health (DrPH) from Harvard. He has worked in several public institutions in Chile, including the Ministry of Economy, the Budget Office and the Ministry of Health. Currently, he is an associate researcher at the Public Health Center Program of the Universidad de Santiago, a member of the Global Long-Term Care Network of the World Health Organization, and an independent consultant on issues related to public policies, health policies, and public health. Pablo is the author of various publications, mainly in the areas of health systems, health financing, aging, and long-term care.

ABOUT THE CONTRIBUTORS

Ahmed Saleh Al Awlaqi is a healthcare leader with experience in project management strategy, policy making and problem solving. He holds a Master in Healthcare Management (Royal College of Surgeons in Ireland), a Master in Health Economics (Université Paris-Sorbonne Abu Dhabi), a Doctoral in Medicine (MD) degree (University of Saarland-Homburg), and Doctoral in Business Administration (DBA) (University of Liverpool). He is part of Mckinsey Company Transformation process with multi tasked integrated Projects and works as Associate Professor at the Université Paris-Sorbonne Abu Dhabi. He was part of previous projects such as IBM Watson Oncology Project in cooperation between Daman-Mubadala, Thiqa Patient support with homecare site visit, Focused behavior Analysis Project for outlier Physicians and Final DRG onsite case manager for efficiency.

Kofi Awuviry-Newton is a social worker by profession and social gerontologist with a broad range of research speciality including healthy ageing, care and caring, social work, disability and functioning. Kofi recently completed his PhD in Gerontology and Geriatrics from The University of Newcastle, and an author of care needs related research papers among older adults in Ghana. His research focuses on the use of interpretative phenomenological analysis (IPA) and other qualitative analysis methods to understand the lived experience of older adults living with functional difficulties and lived experience of caregivers of older peoples.

Julie Byles is Global Innovations Chair in Responsive Transitions in Health and Ageing, Director of the Research Centre for Generational Health and Ageing, and a Director of the Australian Longitudinal Study on Women's Health. As a Fellow and Life Member of the Australian Association of Gerontology, Professor Byles' research interests in ageing include the role of health services, preventive activities, and treatments in maintaining the quality of life for older people. Professor Byles is also Head of the International Longevity Centre – Australia, and Chair of the International Association of Gerontology (Asia Oceania) Social Research and Planning sub-committee.

Judy Feder is a professor of public policy and former dean of what is now Georgetown University's McCourt School of Public Policy. A political scientist by training, she is a nationally-recognized leader in health policy and long-term care policy. Her scholarship at Georgetown University and the Urban Institute led to her election to the National Academy of Medicine. She has also served in senior policy positions in the Congress and the US Department of Health and Human Services; as former chair and board member of AcademyHealth and former board member of the National Academy of Social Insurance; and is a member of the Center for American Progress Action Fund Board and of the Hamilton Project's Advisory Council. In 2006 and 2008, Judy was the Democratic nominee for Congress in Virginia's 10th congressional district. Judy is a political scientist, with a B.A. from Brandeis University, and a master's and PhD from Harvard University.

Emmanuel González-Bautista is an epidemiologist graduated with honors from the Master´s degree in Science in Epidemiology at the National Institute of Public Health in Mexico (INSP, 2015). He is a Medical Doctor from the Autonomous University of the State of Mexico (UAEMex, 2010). He has worked for the Pan American Health Organization / World Health Organization (PAHO/WHO, 2013-2019) in Washington DC and Geneva. He has delivered several workshops in Latin America and the Caribbean for national health systems strengthening through data analysis. Currently, he is a PhD student at the Federal University of Toulouse III in France (2019-2022), with a thesis on the metrics of intrinsic capacity in the context of Integrated Care for Older People (ICOPE). His publications include one book chapter about the Epidemiology of Non-communicable diseases and several peer-reviewed articles on the health of older adults and health over the life course.

Luis Miguel Francisco Gutiérrez-Robledo is an internal medicine specialist who became a geriatrician in France where he worked as assistant professor at the University of Grenoble. Later, he pursued his studies at the University of Paris VII on the biology of aging, receiving his Ph.D. in Public Health from the University of Bordeaux. He has served in the faculty of the National University of Mexico School of Medicine, since 1994 as head of the geriatric medicine specialty program. He founded the Department of Geriatrics at the National Institute of Medical Sciences in 1989 and was its head until January 2009 when he was appointed founder Director General of the National Institute of Geriatrics, position he still holds. He is member of the National Academies of Medicine of Mexico and France. His research agenda focuses on the epidemiology of aging. He has served in various national and global committees including the Advisory Committee at the International Association of Gerontology and Geriatrics, and the World Health Organization; and in the editorial boards of several specialty journals. He has more than 300 publications among books and scientific papers.

Mariana López Ortega holds a PhD in Public Health and Policy from the London School of Hygiene and Tropical Medicine (2010) and Master of Public Policy from the University of Chicago (1997). Since November 2009, she has been working in the Research Department at the National Institute of Geriatrics. She has worked in social and economic analysis of health issues and public health research for over 20 years. Currently, her lines of research in aging and older adults include disability and care dependency, Long-Term Care, social support systems for older adults, social and economic determinants of aging, the value of unpaid care, as well as policies and models of care for older adults.

Fatih Cemil Ozbugday is associate professor of economics at Ankara Yıldırım Beyazit University, in the capital city, Ankara, Turkey. He received his B.Sc. degree in Business Administration from Başkent University, and holds a Master of Arts in Economics (Bilkent University), and a Master of Science degree in International Economics and Finance, as well as a Research Master's degree in Economics from Tilburg University. From 2009 to 2013, he was a Ph.D. researcher at Tilburg University. Dr. Ozbugday's primary research area is industrial organization, applied microeconomics, health economics, and energy economics. His recent academic work focuses on long-term care and resource efficiency. He is a board member of the UNESCO National Commission of Turkey (UTMK) and the head of the Expert Committee for Sustainable Development 2030 Goals.

Mi Sook Song is a professor at college of nursing in AJOU university in South Korea where she is majoring in gerontology and community health care system design for 32 years. Most of her research was performed with empirical data of vulnerable populations in the public sector, based on visiting nursing centers delegated from four local governments for nearly two decades. One of her main achievements was developing a model of customized health care management system, which was finally implemented nationwide in 2007. Recently, her research has been focused on generating evidence for policy-making in order to improve Korean long-term care insurance system.

Hyunjong Song is an associated professor of the Department of Health Policy and Management, College of Health Sciences at Sangji University in South Korea. Her research focuses on the development of community health promotion programs and evaluation of the effectiveness of healthcare and long-term care systems with empirical data and large healthcare databases. She worked as an associate research fellow in Korea Institute of Health and Social Affairs (KIHASA) and as head of the payment system research team in Health Insurance Review and Assessment Service (HIRA). She is a Long-Term Care Insurance Benefit Review Board member and an Advisory Committee Member of Long-term Care Institution Quality Evaluation in National Health Insurance Service (NHIS). Also, she is an Establishment Committee Member of Health Plan and Advisory Committee Member of Emergency Medicine in Korean Ministry of Health and Welfare.

Eduardo Sosa-Tinoco is Master in Public Health and Aging and specialist in Geriatrics and Internal Medicine from the National Autonomous University of Mexico and the National Institute of Medical Sciences and Nutrition Salvador Zubiran. Specialist Physician attached to the Teaching and Outreach Direction, accredited Competencies Trainer and Evaluator of the Certification and Evaluation Entity of the National Institute of Geriatrics (Mexico).

Katherine Swartz is formally retired as Professor of Health Economics and Policy at the Harvard T. H. Chan School of Public Health and is Visiting Professor at Duke University's Sanford School of Public Policy. For more than a dozen years, she has taught a seminar on health policy issues for an aging population. She also is known for her research on health insurance markets. She is a member of the National Academy of Medicine, the National Academy of Social Insurance, and was President of the Association for Public Policy Analysis and Management in 2009. For her work explaining why many Americans are without health insurance, she was the 1991 recipient of the David Kershaw Award for research done before the age of 40 that has had a significant impact on public policy. An economist, she has a BS from the Massachusetts Institute of Technology and a PhD from the University of Wisconsin.

Meredith Tavener is leader in qualitative research at the University of Newcastle, and an award-winning educator. She is recognised nationally and internationally for her innovative qualitative approaches in health research, and her research speciality areas include healthy ageing, men's cancer experiences, recovery after stroke and women's retirement. Dr Tavener is a Fellow of the Australasian Association of Gerontology and member of the International Longevity Centre - Australian chapter.

Abdullah Tirgil is assistant professor in the Department of Public Finance at the Faculty of Political Sciences at Ankara Yıldırım Beyazıt University. Abdullah received a B.Sc. in Management Information Systems, a MA in Economics and MS in Mathematics specialized in Statistics at Western Illinois University, and a Ph.D. in Applied Economics at Northeastern University. His research interests lie in the areas of health economics, labor economics, and applied microeconomics. Abdullah has published several articles in international journals related to the efficiency changes in long-term care, health care utilization of low-income households, out-of-pocket health care expenditures of the most disadvantaged groups in a middle-income country context, and the effects of anti-tobacco policies on tobacco consumption.

Kylie Wales is an occupational therapist and researcher at the University of Newcastle. Kylie's research is reimagining how we assess clients' individual occupational therapy needs, helping to improve their safety and life outcomes. Kylie focuses on exploring how better assessment helps inform occupational therapy practice, allowing for individualized therapy plans, focused service delivery and in turn, cost-effective practice. Kylie's research insights are sought-after. A recent systematic review titled "Functional Assessments Used by Occupational Therapists with Older Adults at Risk of Activity and Participation Limitations" was in the top one percent of PLOS ONE's most downloaded articles.

INDEX

A

accreditation, 153, 177, 178, 183, 206, 235, 236, 241, 242
activities of daily living (ADL), 1, 16, 26, 34, 35, 42, 46, 122, 137, 174, 176, 180, 182, 188, 193, 209, 219, 223, 225
aging, ix, xi, xii, xiii, 2, 5, 6, 8, 9, 10, 13, 14, 15, 20, 22, 23, 24, 27, 28, 30, 31, 47, 50, 61, 65, 68, 70, 101, 102, 105, 106, 108, 112, 113, 115, 137, 139, 140, 142, 145, 147, 170, 173, 187, 191, 198, 203, 204, 207, 209, 211, 212, 217, 218, 230, 231, 233, 238, 240, 242, 245, 249, 250, 251, 252
aging in place, xiii, 142, 233
assisted living facilities, 82, 90

B

benefits, xii, xiii, 10, 11, 17, 39, 43, 44, 46, 76, 77, 81, 82, 96, 99, 100, 101, 102, 103, 124, 125, 129, 130, 146, 148, 149, 150, 164, 172, 186, 188, 193, 202, 222, 224, 225, 227, 229, 231, 233, 234, 238

C

CARES Act, 93, 94
case fatality rate, 90, 91
catastrophic public long-term care insurance, 100
Centers for Medicare and Medicaid Services, 77, 86, 106, 108
certified home health agency, 80
certified nursing assistants, 84, 88
chain-affiliated, 89
chains, 88, 109, 110
community spread, 91, 104

D

dementia, 16, 28, 47, 51, 52, 53, 54, 55, 61, 66, 68, 69, 147, 180, 191, 193, 212, 220, 222, 224, 225, 226, 229, 232, 234, 238, 240, 241
dementia prevalence, 52, 54, 61, 69, 220

demographic, v, ix, xi, xiii, 1, 2, 3, 6, 8, 9, 10, 14, 15, 18, 19, 20, 22, 25, 27, 28, 29, 47, 48, 61, 77, 123, 133, 169, 173, 185, 186, 218
demographic and epidemiologic transitions, 9, 29
demographic and epidemiological changes, xi, 14
demographic and epidemiological transitions, 1, 8, 10, 18
demographic change, v, ix, 2, 6, 61, 169
demographic transition, 2, 3, 6, 8, 19, 22, 185, 218
Department of Veterans Affairs, 80, 83
direct-care workers, 84, 85, 96

E

eligibility, 34, 46, 76, 81, 82, 83, 101, 106, 108, 112, 146, 148, 163, 164, 222, 227
environmental, 22, 121, 123, 134, 136, 141, 171
environmental factors, 123, 134
environmental impediments, 121
environmental modifications, 136
expenditure, 9, 29, 68, 156, 157, 162, 166, 210
extended family, 38, 124, 126, 128, 140

F

factors, xii, 25, 27, 28, 47, 57, 68, 70, 86, 88, 91, 92, 118, 121, 123, 124, 127, 128, 134, 136, 137, 138, 141, 145, 162, 163, 166, 185, 186, 189, 209, 240, 241, 242
family caregiving, 66, 80, 140, 202, 234
Federal Medical Assistance Percentages (FMAPs), 94, 95
federal poverty level, 81, 85, 96
fertility rate, 2, 29, 118, 119, 175, 186, 219
financing, vii, xii, xiii, 10, 16, 18, 21, 26, 27, 33, 45, 46, 65, 66, 67, 74, 75, 78, 80, 93, 100, 101, 102, 108, 136, 143, 145, 146, 148, 149, 150, 152, 154, 155, 156, 157, 158, 159, 161, 162, 163, 164, 165, 167, 168, 169, 170, 174, 178, 185, 188, 192, 193, 194, 206, 212, 215, 226, 227, 230, 245
financing of LTC, xii, 16, 18, 27, 74, 78, 155, 163
for-profit, 82, 88, 110, 178, 179, 180
functional abilities, 18

G

Germany, 13, 16, 20, 22, 23, 45, 52, 58, 136, 147, 148, 149, 150, 163, 164, 169, 170, 241
Ghana, vii, xi, xii, 117, 118, 120, 121, 122, 123, 124, 125, 126, 127, 128, 129, 130, 131, 132, 133, 134, 135, 136, 137, 138, 139, 140, 141, 142, 247
Ghana National Ageing Policy, 133
Government Accountability Office (GAO), 86, 87, 97, 109
gray market, 85

H

HCBS, 81, 82, 86, 95, 98
health system, xii, 6, 8, 10, 17, 22, 155, 165, 169, 171, 172, 190, 209, 212, 213, 240, 242, 245, 249
healthcare, xiii, 8, 18, 26, 91, 109, 111, 129, 130, 133, 134, 135, 143, 144, 146, 147, 148, 150, 151, 152, 153, 154, 155, 156, 159, 161, 162, 165, 167, 169, 170, 171, 172, 190, 247, 251
healthcare financing, 144, 146, 148, 153, 154, 155, 162, 165
healthcare sector, 152, 154, 155, 165

healthcare system, 130, 144, 150, 151, 155, 165
healthcare workers, 91, 109, 111, 151
HEROES bill, 95
holistic, 121, 123, 124, 135, 136, 140
holistic intervention, 136
holistic perspective, 121, 123
home and community-based services, 81, 95
home and community-based settings, 80
home health aides, 84, 85
home health services, 79
home-based care, 26, 32, 33, 34, 36, 37, 38, 42
housekeeping and companion services, 84

I

informal care, 12, 19, 24, 26, 36, 48, 55, 56, 57, 59, 62, 63, 66, 68, 70, 77, 128, 157, 162, 181, 189, 207, 212
informal care-giving, 77
institutional settings, 76
instrumental activities of daily living (IADL), 174, 176, 219
insurance, xii, xiii, 16, 19, 20, 22, 23, 30, 45, 65, 66, 74, 75, 76, 78, 79, 80, 94, 96, 102, 103, 104, 105, 107, 111, 129, 130, 131, 140, 147, 149, 150, 154, 155, 156, 157, 158, 159, 160, 161, 163, 164, 166, 192, 217, 221, 222, 226, 227, 228, 234, 236, 240, 241, 242, 243, 248, 251, 252
intermediate care facilities, 114
intermediate care providers, 83
intervention, 130, 135, 136, 207, 233, 237
intrinsic capacities, 120

J

Japan, 13, 20, 23, 27, 58, 67, 68, 138, 147, 148, 150, 163, 164, 167, 195, 213, 218, 233, 236, 239, 241
Jobs and Growth Tax Relief Reconciliation Act, 95

K

Korea, viii, xi, xiii, 13, 16, 20, 22, 23, 27, 36, 45, 58, 68, 147, 163, 164, 217, 218, 219, 220, 221, 222, 224, 225, 226, 228, 229, 230, 231, 233, 234, 235, 236, 237, 238, 239, 240, 241, 242, 250, 251

L

labor force, 9, 38, 50, 55, 56, 57, 61, 62, 162, 175, 238
labor market, 11, 48, 55, 62, 186, 190, 193
Latin America, 4, 24, 193, 249
licensed practical nurses, 84, 88
life expectancy, 7, 29, 74, 103, 118, 119, 120, 144, 168, 175, 214, 217, 219, 220, 240
Livelihood Empowerment against Poverty (LEAP), 129, 138
long-term care (LTC) needs, v, vii, ix, x, xi, xii, 2, 9, 14, 15, 16, 17, 36, 64, 66, 70, 76, 77, 78, 81, 95, 96, 98, 101, 117, 118, 120, 121, 122, 133, 135, 136, 143, 148, 155, 162, 165, 175, 223, 233, 239
Long-Term Care Insurance (LTCI), viii, 20, 68, 80, 82, 167, 170, 217, 221, 222, 224, 225, 226, 227, 228, 229, 230, 231, 232, 233, 234, 235, 236, 237, 238, 239, 251
long-term services and supports, 76, 167, 168
LTC financing, x, 16, 94, 145, 146, 148, 149, 150, 155, 159, 161, 162, 163, 164, 165
LTC insurance, 27, 30, 33, 47, 63, 64, 107, 147, 148, 149, 150, 159, 160
LTC system, x, xi, xii, xiii, 1, 10, 11, 12, 13, 14, 15, 16, 17, 18, 19, 28, 32, 34, 43, 45,

135, 145, 146, 147, 148, 174, 177, 181, 184, 185, 186, 188, 190, 191, 192, 193, 194, 195, 196, 198, 199, 200, 204, 205, 207, 208, 239
LTCI beneficiaries, 225, 230, 231, 232
LTCI benefits, 224
LTCI eligibility, 222, 238, 239
LTCI expenditure, 229, 231, 232
LTCI services, 231, 236, 238, 239
LTCI system, 217, 221, 232, 234, 238

M

Medicaid, xii, 17, 20, 75, 76, 80, 81, 82, 83, 84, 85, 86, 87, 89, 90, 91, 92, 93, 94, 95, 96, 97, 98, 99, 101, 104, 105, 107, 108, 109, 110, 112, 113, 114, 115, 235
medically needy, 81
Medicare, 17, 20, 22, 78, 79, 80, 81, 83, 84, 85, 86, 87, 88, 89, 97, 98, 99, 100, 101, 102, 106, 107, 111, 112, 168, 235
Medicare Advantage, 79
Medicare Part B, 79
Medicare-certified home health agencies, 84
Mexican Health and Aging Study (MHAS), 174, 176, 183
multifactorial, 118, 121, 134, 136

N

National Ageing Policy, 132, 133, 135, 139
National Health Insurance Scheme (NHIS), 129, 130, 131, 135, 139, 140, 222, 223, 224, 225, 228, 229, 232, 233, 234, 235, 237, 238, 239, 240, 241, 243, 251
National Institute of Geriatrics (INGER), 173, 177, 189, 196, 197, 198, 199, 201, 207, 211, 249, 250, 251
needs, v, ix, x, 1, 8, 9, 10, 11, 14, 15, 16, 18, 19, 20, 21, 26, 31, 34, 37, 43, 65, 68, 73, 75, 76, 78, 80, 85, 87, 89, 94, 96, 101, 103, 114, 117, 118, 120, 121, 123, 124, 125, 126, 128, 129, 130, 131, 132, 133, 134, 135, 136, 138, 139, 143, 144, 145, 147, 150, 151, 152, 153, 155, 161, 162, 163, 164, 165, 169, 170, 175, 176, 180, 184, 185, 194, 199, 200, 202, 210, 221, 223, 224, 226, 229, 230, 231, 232, 233, 234, 238, 239, 240, 247, 253
needs assessment, 163, 223, 233
non-profit, 82, 88, 89, 178, 179, 180, 182, 187
nursing home industry, 87, 92, 97
nursing homes, 20, 26, 27, 29, 34, 35, 36, 38, 40, 41, 46, 50, 63, 64, 65, 66, 73, 74, 76, 77, 78, 81, 82, 83, 85, 86, 87, 88, 89, 90, 91, 92, 93, 96, 97, 98, 99, 101, 104, 105, 106, 107, 108, 109, 111, 112, 113, 114, 128, 132, 147, 157, 159, 187, 194, 195, 198, 213, 225, 235, 236, 237, 241
nursing staffing levels, 86

P

pathways, 81, 190, 191, 215
personal care assistant, 84
personal protective equipment, 88, 91, 112
person-centered care, 191, 238
perspective, xi, 6, 12, 13, 14, 20, 51, 73, 75, 121, 134, 137, 140, 194, 205, 241
plans for infection prevention and control, 87
post-acute care, 79, 80
prevalence, 8, 9, 28, 47, 50, 52, 61, 122, 138, 141, 173, 174, 176, 209, 220, 229, 237
private equity investors, 88
private long-term care insurance, 80, 111
private-pay, 83, 84, 89, 90
private-pay aides, 84
profit margins, 89

Q

quality deficiencies, 86

R

reciprocity, 124, 125, 142
registered nurses, 84
rehabilitation, 29, 30, 34, 35, 36, 38, 39, 42, 43, 45, 46, 79, 136, 157, 180, 187, 223
residential and day care, 39
residential care, 26, 30, 36, 39, 42, 43, 44, 50, 53, 60, 74, 77, 83, 85, 178
residential care facilities, 74, 77, 83, 85
residential facilities, 82, 83, 157
resource allocation, 145, 146, 155, 161, 162, 165, 185

S

sector, 11, 16, 60, 63, 65, 130, 131, 140, 143, 145, 147, 149, 151, 152, 153, 154, 155, 157, 158, 159, 160, 163, 165, 166, 178, 181, 182, 187, 190, 193, 194, 197, 198, 201, 205, 208, 234, 250
self-employed aides, 84
services, iv, ix, xi, xii, xiii, 2, 9, 10, 11, 12, 13, 14, 15, 16, 17, 18, 19, 20, 24, 26, 29, 30, 31, 32, 33, 34, 35, 36, 37, 38, 39, 40, 41, 42, 43, 44, 45, 46, 59, 60, 61, 63, 65, 66, 67, 68, 69, 70, 76, 77, 79, 81, 82, 83, 84, 86, 87, 89, 93, 94, 99, 101, 103,106, 107, 110, 111, 113, 114, 115, 116, 129, 132, 134, 135, 143, 144, 145, 146, 147, 148, 150, 151, 152, 153, 154, 156, 157, 158, 159, 160, 161, 162, 163, 165, 168, 169, 172, 174, 175, 177, 178, 179, 180, 181, 182, 183, 184, 185, 186, 188, 190, 193, 194, 195, 196, 197, 198, 199, 200, 201, 204, 205, 207, 214, 215, 217, 224, 225, 226, 227, 230, 231, 232, 233, 234, 235, 236, 237, 238, 239, 240, 241, 242, 248
shared responsibility, 100
skilled nursing, 79, 82, 83, 84
skilled nursing facilities, 82, 83
skilled nursing facility, 79
social insurance program, 74, 94, 100, 101, 102, 103
Social Insurance System, 99
social security, xi, 1, 6, 8, 10, 11, 12, 14, 18, 20, 24, 33, 70, 81, 85, 100, 101, 102, 129, 131, 139, 140, 184, 191, 193, 194, 199, 215
Social Security and National Insurance Trust, 129, 131
Special Focus Facilities, 87, 98, 107
staffing, 83, 86, 87, 88, 92, 96, 97, 98, 108, 110, 112, 225, 226, 236, 238, 241
staffing-to-resident ratios, 92
Standard Care Plan, 224, 231, 233, 234, 238
state and local revenue shortfalls, 93
sub-Saharan Africa, 4, 117, 118, 119, 120, 125, 140, 142
sustaining LTC, 118
system, iv, viii, xi, xii, xiii, 6, 9, 10, 11, 12, 13, 15, 16, 17, 18, 23, 28, 29, 32, 33, 45, 47, 48, 63, 65, 70, 73, 74, 75, 98, 99, 103, 114, 116, 124, 126, 128, 130, 132, 146, 147, 150, 153, 159, 161, 163, 164, 166, 167, 172, 173, 174, 177, 184, 185, 186, 188, 189, 191, 193, 194, 195, 196, 198, 199, 202, 204, 205, 209, 213, 217, 222, 223, 227, 228, 233, 234, 235, 236, 237, 238, 240, 241, 250, 251

T

tasks of daily life, 76
tasks of daily living, 76, 79

technology, 167, 180, 190, 193, 195, 202, 207, 208, 252
Turkey, vii, xi, 25, 26, 28, 29, 30, 31, 32, 33, 34, 35, 36, 37, 38, 41, 42, 43, 44, 45, 46, 47, 48, 49, 50, 51, 52, 53, 55, 56, 57, 58, 59, 61, 62, 63, 64, 65, 68, 69, 250

U

unpaid LTC, 77

W

waivers, 82
workers, 26, 28, 48, 63, 64, 85, 89, 90, 91, 92, 96, 103, 109, 115, 123, 131, 135, 141, 152, 155, 158, 159, 181, 187, 215, 225, 226, 227, 234, 236, 238